# Pocket Manual of General Thoracic Surgery

D1553525

Amin Madani • Lorenzo Ferri
Andrew Seely

Editors

# Pocket Manual of General Thoracic Surgery

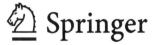 Springer

*Editors*
Amin Madani, M.D.
McGill University
Montreal, QC, Canada

Lorenzo Ferri, M.D., Ph.D.,
  F.A.C.S., F.R.C.S.C.
McGill University
Montreal, QC, Canada

Andrew Seely, M.D., Ph.D.,
  F.R.C.S.C.
The Ottawa Hospital – General
  Campus
University of Ottawa
Ottawa, ON, Canada

ISBN 978-3-319-17496-9      ISBN 978-3-319-17497-6   (eBook)
DOI 10.1007/978-3-319-17497-6

Library of Congress Control Number: 2015941503

Springer Cham Heidelberg New York Dordrecht London

Printed on acid-free paper

Springer International Publishing AG Switzerland is part of Springer
Science+Business Media (www.springer.com)

# Preface

The field of general thoracic surgery has undergone significant changes over the past decade as new scientific literature and paradigms of patient care are continuously introduced. Despite these advancements and complexities in the management of thoracic patients, there are very few educational tools available to trainees that can synthesize the vast collection of information into a concise format. While there are already various outstanding textbooks in general thoracic surgery available, there is a need for a quick reference and evidence-based manual that is readily accessible to help trainees manage patients effectively in the clinic, operating room, ward, intensive care unit, and emergency department.

This manual is organized into 9 chapters providing a concise, yet inclusive list of the most common pathologies seen in thoracic surgery: preoperative evaluation, perioperative care, lungs and airways (divided into three separate sections to cover the vast number of topics), pleural disorders, mediastinal disorders, chest wall disorders, thoracic trauma, and benign and malignant esophageal disorders. The content of each chapter was specifically structured so that the handbook can be a high-yield reference that includes numerous management algorithms, flow diagrams, tables, and images. Unlike a comprehensive textbook, paragraphs are kept at a minimum and the written material is presented using lists and bullet points to facilitate learning and retention. More importantly, an enormous amount of effort was dedicated to keep the content evidence-based and to highlight the controversies in the field.

Finally, we would like to thank the contributors, without whom this book would not be possible.

Montreal, QC, Canada              Amin Madani, M.D.
Montreal, QC, Canada      Lorenzo Ferri, M.D., Ph.D.,
                                          F.A.C.S., F.R.C.S.C.
Ottawa, ON, Canada    Andrew Seely, M.D., Ph.D., F.R.C.S.C.
October 2014

# Disclaimer

The content presented herein is provided as a basic guideline for approaching selected pathologies in general thoracic surgery. The intention of this book is to serve as an adjunct to other educational resources for trainees in order to assist them with the management of their patients. The authors of this book make no claims regarding the handbook's educational value and/or contribution to performance on any certification examinations (high stakes or otherwise). Finally, while the information presented herein is believed to be factual and as true as possible to date, neither the Publisher nor the authors, contributors, or editors assume any liability for any injury and/or damage to persons or property as a matter of products liability, negligence or otherwise, or from any use of operation of any methods, products, instructions, or ideas contained in the material herein.

# Contents

# Contributors

**Ali Aboalsaud, M.D.** Department of Surgery, McGill University Health Center, Montreal, QC, Canada

**Maria Abou-Khalil** Department of Surgery, McGill University Health Center, Montreal, QC, Canada

**Hussam Alamri, M.D.** Department of Surgery, McGill University Health Center, Montreal, QC, Canada

**Mohammed Al-Mahroos, M.D.** Department of Surgery, McGill University Health Center, Montreal, QC, Canada

**Abdullah Aloraini, M.B.B.S., M.P.H.** Department of Surgery, McGill University Health Center, Montreal, QC, Canada

**Dan L. Deckelbaum, M.D.** Department of Surgery, McGill University Health Center, Montreal, QC, Canada

**Stephen D. Gowing, M.D.** Department of Surgery, McGill University Health Center, Montreal, QC, Canada

**Amin Madani, M.D.** Department of Surgery, McGill University Health Center, Montreal, QC, Canada

**Sara Najmeh, B.Sc., M.D.** Department of Surgery, McGill University Health Center, Montreal, QC, Canada

**Etienne St-Louis, M.D., C.M.** Department of Surgery, McGill University Health Center, Montreal, QC, Canada

**Monisha Sudarshan, M.D., M.P.H.** Department of Surgery, McGill University Health Center, Montreal, QC, Canada

# Chapter 1
# Preoperative Evaluation of the Thoracic Patient

**Amin Madani**

- One of the most important skills a thoracic surgeon must master is the determination of *operability*, namely, a patient's ability to tolerate thoracic surgery—most commonly pulmonary resection.
- Thoracic surgical patients tend to have reduced baseline cardiopulmonary function due to cigarette smoking, COPD, atherosclerotic cardiovascular disease, and possibly hypertension, diabetes and advanced age, putting them at significant risk of perioperative morbidity and mortality.

  - Mortality risk 2 % after lobectomy; 4–7 % after pneumonectomy.

- The most lethal of perioperative complications after noncardiac thoracic surgery are respiratory and cardiovascular. The preoperative evaluation therefore needs to objectively evaluate such risk factors (Fig. 1.1).

  - One of the principal goals of preoperative evaluation is to balance the benefit of a curative-intent surgical resection and the risks of immediate and long-term postoperative complications.

A. Madani, M.D. (✉)
Department of Surgery, McGill University,
Montreal, QC, Canada
e-mail: amin.madani@mail.mcgill.ca

A. Madani et al. (eds.), *Pocket Manual of General Thoracic Surgery*, DOI 10.1007/978-3-319-17497-6_1,
© Springer International Publishing Switzerland 2015

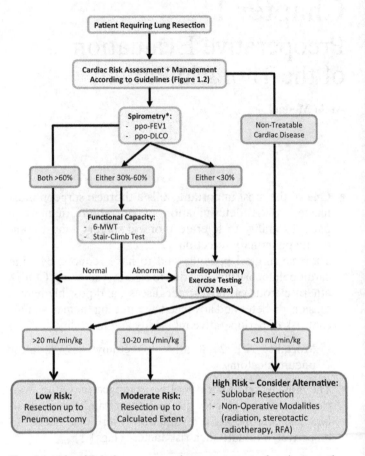

Fig. 1.1. Algorithm for preoperative assessment of patients undergoing lung resection [2].

- While increased perioperative mortality occurs with age >70 (4 vs. 1.4 %, OR 3.6 [95 % CI, 1.4–8.9]) [1], age alone should not be the only determinant of a patient's operability.

# Physiological Consequences of Thoracic Surgery

## General to All Surgery

- Inhaled volatile agents cause changes in diaphragm and chest wall function, creating areas of decreased ventilation, which leads to ventilation to perfusion (V/Q) mismatch and subsequent hypoxemia.

## Specific to Thoracic Surgery

- Postoperative chest wall pain causes:
  - Decreased functional residual capacity (FRC) up to 30–35 % with subsequent atelectasis.
  - Poor cough with inability to clear pulmonary secretion and increased risk of pneumonia.
- Thoracic patients should be evaluated preoperatively to screen for patients at high risk of perioperative complications (Fig. 1.1).

### Pulmonary Resection

- Impaired FEV1.
- Impaired cough.
- Atelectasis.

### Single-Lung Ventilation

- Initially causes 50 % right to left shunt, V/Q mismatch, and hypoxemia [3].
- However, compensatory mechanisms in the atelectatic lung decrease perfusion (hypoxic pulmonary vasoconstriction, manipulation of the lung during surgery, and gravitational force from lateral decubitus position). Shunt fraction therefore decreases to 25 %.
- Can lead to acute lung injury (ALI) or acute respiratory distress syndrome (ARDS). Risk factors include high tidal volume and airway pressure.

- Protective ventilation strategies can decrease injury: low tidal volume ventilation, use of positive end-expiratory pressure (PEEP), and minimizing airway pressure and fraction of inspired oxygen.

**Bronchial Anastomoses**

- Impaired mucociliary clearance and buildup of secretions.

**Proximal Foregut Anastomoses**

- Impaired swallowing and risk of aspiration.

## Mitigation of Cardiopulmonary Adverse Events

- Cigarette smoking: all active smokers should be encouraged to stop at least 2 weeks before surgery (preferably >6 weeks). Patients should be offered counselling, smoking cessation programs, and pharmacologic assistance.
- Estimation of postoperative predicted pulmonary function to assess and stratify risk of pulmonary complications, perioperative morbidity and mortality, and long-term functional disability (Fig. 1.1).
- Identification of cardiac patients in need of medical management or coronary revascularization (Fig. 1.2).
- Preoperative exercise program in all patients.

## Cardiac Assessment

- All noncardiac thoracic surgical patients should undergo a cardiac risk assessment based on history, physical examination and baseline electrocardiogram (EKG), and managed according to the 2014 American College of Cardiology/American Heart Association guidelines (Fig. 1.2) [4].

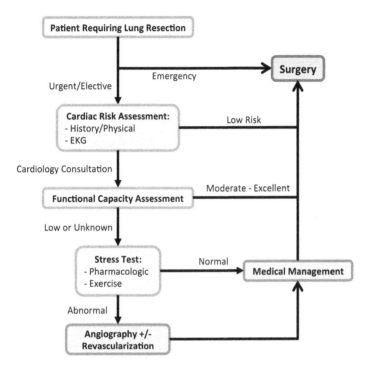

FIG. 1.2. Algorithm for preoperative cardiac assessment of patients undergoing lung resection [4].

- Emergency surgery: proceed to surgery.
- Urgent/elective surgery:

   If patient is suffering from an acute coronary syndrome, they should be managed according to NSTEMI or STEMI clinical practice guidelines and referred to cardiology.

   Evaluate for risk factors of coronary artery disease (CAD) and overall risk of experiencing major adverse cardiac event using risk calculators such as the American College of Surgeons-NSQIP or Revised Cardiac Risk Index. No further testing is needed for patients with low risk (<1 %).

Patients at risk of major adverse cardiac event should be evaluated for functional capacity using an objective scale. No further testing is needed for patients with moderate to excellent functional capacity.

Patients with poor or unknown functional capacity should undergo either pharmacologic or exercise stress testing. Patients with normal stress test can me managed medically and undergo surgery. Patients with abnormal stress test should undergo coronary angiography ± revascularization followed by appropriate medical management prior to proceeding with surgery. Alternatively, a noninvasive surgical approach should be considered (e.g., chemoradiation for malignancy).

- Cardiac testing [4]:

  - Electrocardiogram: indicated in patients with CAD, significant arrhythmia, peripheral arterial disease, cerebrovascular disease or other structural heart diseases. Routine 12-lead EKG is not necessary for asymptomatic patients undergoing low-risk surgical procedures.
  - Echocardiogram: indicated to rule out asymptomatic pulmonary hypertension in patients who may require pneumonectomy, or in patients with suspected impaired cardiac function, heart failure (e.g., dyspnea of unknown origin), CAD or valvular disease. Patients with previous left ventricular (LV) dysfunction, should also be reevaluated if >1 year since the last evaluation.
  - Stress testing: indicated in patients with or at high risk for ischemic heart disease in order to identify patients who may require further medical therapy or coronary revascularization prior to thoracic surgery.
  - Angiogram: indicated to rule out life-threatening coronary stenosis in patients with significantly positive stress tests.

# Pulmonary Function Tests (PFT)

- Indications:
  - Significant baseline airflow obstruction with known obstructive pulmonary disease
  - Significant pleural disease
  - Central lung mass or suspected endobronchial obstruction
  - Prior lung resection

- Not indicated for surgeries without lung resection (e.g., esophagectomy, mediastinoscopy, pleural biopsy or drainage), and in patients without prior history of lung disease, unexplained dyspnea, or functional limitation.

## Baseline Forced Expiratory Volume in 1 Second (FEV1) and Diffusing Capacity of the Lung for Carbon Monoxide (DLCO)

- Most commonly used predictors of postoperative pulmonary reserve.

  - *Neoadjuvant Chemotherapy*: decreases preoperative and increases perioperative DLCO [5]. Patients who undergo neoadjuvant therapy should undergo repeat PFT after the completion of therapy [2].
  - Anemia most common cause of falsely low DLCO. Other factors interfering with the interpretation or accuracy of pulmonary function tests include use of bronchodilators, narcotics, pregnancy, increased intra-abdominal pressure (e.g., gastric distension), fatigue, and other conditions limiting the patient's ability to perform spirometry.

- Mortality <5 % with preoperative FEV1 >1.5 L for lobectomy and >2.0 L or >80 % for pneumonectomy [6].

  - Most patients with FEV1 >60 % will tolerate a lobectomy (morbidity rate 12 %), depending on age and comorbidities [7].

- FEV1 is an independent predictor of pulmonary complications and cardiac complications (OR increases by 1.1 for every 10 % decrease in FEV1) [8].
- DLCO <70 % has been identified as a predictor of mortality and pulmonary complications [9] and may require additional physiologic testing prior to resection (e.g., exercise testing—VO2 Max).

## Predicted Postoperative FEV1 and DLCO (ppo-FEV1, ppo-DLCO)

- Functional pulmonary reserve should be calculated for all patients according to the third edition American College of Chest Physicians guidelines [2].
  - Simple calculation (assumes homogenous distribution of lung function):

    ppo  Value = Baseline × [1 – (Number  of  Resected Segments × 0.0526)]

  - Regional assessment: quantitative radionuclide V/Q scanning (xenon-133) or quantitative CT scanning (subtracts the exact contribution of the lung to be resected).

    ppo Value = Baseline × (1 – proportion of ventilation or perfusion in resected lung)

- Predicted postoperative values underestimate the true functional loss that occurs in the immediate postoperative period (i.e., lung function is markedly lower than what was predicted) [10, 11].

  - The gap between measured and predicted values is greatest on postoperative days 0–6 and eventually decreases (actual FEV1 is 70 % of ppo-FEV1 on postoperative day 1, and 90 % of ppo-FEV1 on postoperative day 7). At 1 month, the measured and predicted values become equal (100 % of ppo-FEV1).

- Ppo-DLCO <40 % shown to be a very strong predictor of postoperative complications [12].
    - OR 1.12 per 10-point decrease [13].
- Patients with ppo-FEV1 <40 % have a high risk of perioperative mortality (5–10 %) and cardiopulmonary complications (30–50 %). This high-risk designation must be interpreted by the surgeon and patient together to determine optimal management.
- 10 % increase in postoperative respiratory complications for every 5 % decrease in ppo-FEV1 and ppo-DLCO [14].
- Most studies suggest that patients can undergo surgery with ppo lung function as low as 30 %, as long as they demonstrate acceptable exercise capacity.
- Latest guidelines recommend using ppo-FEV1 and ppo-DLCO cutoffs at 60 %[2]:
    - Both >60 %: no further testing required; patient can proceed to surgery and tolerate resection up to pnuemonectomy with minimal risk of cardiopulmonary complications or death.
    - Either <60 %: further testing required to assess functional capacity.

## Functional Capacity and Cardiopulmonary Exercise Testing (CPET)

- Indicated for patients with ppo-FEV1 or ppo-DLCO <60 %.
    - 30–60 %: low-technology exercise testing (6-min Walk Test (6-MWT), stair-climb test) screening, followed by CPET if abnormal.
    - <30 %: patient should directly undergo CPET.

*Low-Technology Noninvasive Tests for Functional Capacity: 6-min Walk Test (6-MWT), Stair-Climb Test*

- 6-MWT:
  - Correlates with pulmonary function, health-related quality of life, VO2 Max and mortality. Used to predict response to therapy and prognosis.
  - Distance <350 m associated with increased mortality in patients with COPD, heart failure and pulmonary arterial hypertension.
  - Preoperative evaluation [15]:

    >550 m: does not require CPET.
    <400 m: should undergo further evaluation of VO2 Max.
    428–562 m: depends on patient factors and magnitude of surgery.

  - Desaturation during the test is a strong risk factor for mortality in patients with interstitial lung disease (fourfold) [16]. Patients with desaturation >4 % during exercise have increased risk of perioperative morbidity [17].
  - Minimal clinically important difference (smallest change in outcome that is meaningful to patients): 54–80 m [18].
  - Varies with age, gender, height, and weight [19].

- Stair-Climb Test:
  - >22 m: satisfactory test; patient may undergo anatomic lung resection (very low risk postoperative mortality).
  - <22 m: abnormal; patient should undergo further evaluation of VO2 Max (<12 m: 15–20 % mortality) [20].
  - General rule-of-thumb: >5 flights of stairs for pneumonectomy; >2 flights of stairs for a lobectomy.

## CPET: Maximal Oxygen Consumption (VO2 Max) Testing

- Indicated for patients with either ppo-FEV1 or ppo-DLCO <30 %, or patients with abnormal 6-MWT or stair-climb tests.
- VO2 Max <15 mL/min/kg associated with increased peri-operative risk (mortality 7–20 %).
- VO2 Max <10 mL/min/kg associated with very high risk (mortality 26–50 %).
- VO2 Max >20 mL/min/kg associated with low risk.
- *Ppo-VO2 Max* (*Predicted Postoperative VO2 Max*): <10 mL/min/kg (<35 % predicted) also associated with high postoperative mortality [21].

# Arterial Blood Gas

- Resting hypercapnea ($pCO_2 > 45$ mmHg) is normally due to alveolar hypoventilation and remains a major concern for pulmonary resection. Historically quoted as an exclusion criterion for lung resection.
- Hypercapnea has not been shown to have a strong relationship with perioperative complications or mortality following major lung resection [22, 23]. Therefore, it is not currently considered a contraindication to lung resection by itself.

# References

1. Damhuis RA, Schutte PR. Resection rates and postoperative mortality in 7,899 patients with lung cancer. Eur Respir J. 1996;9(1):7–10.
2. Brunelli A, et al. Physiologic evaluation of the patient with lung cancer being considered for resectional surgery: Diagnosis and management of lung cancer, 3rd ed: American College of Chest Physicians evidence-based clinical practice guidelines. Chest. 2013;143(5 Suppl):e166S–90.

3. Karzai W, Schwarzkopf K. Hypoxemia during one-lung ventilation: prediction, prevention, and treatment. Anesthesiology. 2009;110(6):1402–11.
4. Fleisher LA, et al. 2014 ACC/AHA guideline on perioperative cardiovascular evaluation and management of patients undergoing noncardiac surgery: a report of the American College of Cardiology/American Heart Association Task Force on practice guidelines. J Am Coll Cardiol. 2014;64(22):e77–137.
5. Matsubara Y, Takeda S, Mashimo T. Risk stratification for lung cancer surgery: impact of induction therapy and extended resection. Chest. 2005;128(5):3519–25.
6. Brunelli A, et al. ERS/ESTS clinical guidelines on fitness for radical therapy in lung cancer patients (surgery and chemoradiotherapy). Eur Respir J. 2009;34(1):17–41.
7. Berry MF, et al. Pulmonary function tests do not predict pulmonary complications after thoracoscopic lobectomy. Ann Thorac Surg. 2010;89(4):1044–51. discussion 1051-2.
8. Ferguson MK, Siddique J, Karrison T. Modeling major lung resection outcomes using classification trees and multiple imputation techniques. Eur J Cardiothorac Surg. 2008;34(5):1085–9.
9. Ferguson MK, et al. Diffusing capacity predicts morbidity and mortality after pulmonary resection. J Thorac Cardiovasc Surg. 1988;96(6):894–900.
10. Varela G, et al. Predicted versus observed FEV1 in the immediate postoperative period after pulmonary lobectomy. Eur J Cardiothorac Surg. 2006;30(4):644–8.
11. Brunelli A, et al. Predicted versus observed FEV1 and DLCO after major lung resection: a prospective evaluation at different postoperative periods. Ann Thorac Surg. 2007;83(3):1134–9.
12. Brunelli A, et al. Carbon monoxide lung diffusion capacity improves risk stratification in patients without airflow limitation: evidence for systematic measurement before lung resection. Eur J Cardiothorac Surg. 2006;29(4):567–70.
13. Ferguson MK, et al. Pulmonary complications after lung resection in the absence of chronic obstructive pulmonary disease: the predictive role of diffusing capacity. J Thorac Cardiovasc Surg. 2009;138(6):1297–302.
14. Alam N, et al. Incidence and risk factors for lung injury after lung cancer resection. Ann Thorac Surg. 2007;84(4):1085–91. discussion 1091.
15. Sinclair RC, et al. Validity of the 6 min walk test in prediction of the anaerobic threshold before major non-cardiac surgery. Br J Anaesth. 2012;108(1):30–5.

16. Lama VN, et al. Prognostic value of desaturation during a 6-minute walk test in idiopathic interstitial pneumonia. Am J Respir Crit Care Med. 2003;168(9):1084–90.
17. Ninan M, et al. Standardized exercise oximetry predicts postpneumonectomy outcome. Ann Thorac Surg. 1997;64(2):328–32. discussion 332-3.
18. Wise RA, Brown CD. Minimal clinically important differences in the six-minute walk test and the incremental shuttle walking test. COPD. 2005;2(1):125–9.
19. Rasekaba T, et al. The six-minute walk test: a useful metric for the cardiopulmonary patient. Intern Med J. 2009;39(8):495–501.
20. Brunelli A, et al. Performance at symptom-limited stair-climbing test is associated with increased cardiopulmonary complications, mortality, and costs after major lung resection. Ann Thorac Surg. 2008;86(1):240–7. discussion 247-8.
21. Bolliger CT, et al. Lung scanning and exercise testing for the prediction of postoperative performance in lung resection candidates at increased risk for complications. Chest. 1995;108(2):341–8.
22. Kearney DJ, et al. Assessment of operative risk in patients undergoing lung resection. Importance of predicted pulmonary function. Chest. 1994;105(3):753–9.
23. Harpole DH, et al. Prospective analysis of pneumonectomy: risk factors for major morbidity and cardiac dysrhythmias. Ann Thorac Surg. 1996;61(3):977–82.

# Chapter 2
# Operative and Postoperative Considerations

**Hussam Alamri**

## Intraoperative Considerations

- Three main options for lung isolation during single-lung ventilation exist:
    1. Endobronchial intubation
    2. Bronchial blocker
    3. Double lumen tube (DLT)

- After sedation, diagnostic bronchoscopy is performed to identify any anatomical or pathological findings that might affect lung isolation strategies and confirm anatomy of planned bronchial resection. Final positioning of lung isolation tubes or blockers should be confirmed with fiber-optic bronchoscopy and subsequently repeated after patient re-positioning and when necessary during a thoracic operative procedure.

H. Alamri, M.D. (✉)
Department of Surgery, McGill University, 1650 Cedar Avenue, Montreal, QC, Canada H3G 1A4
e-mail: hussam.alamri@mail.mcgill.ca

A. Madani et al. (eds.), *Pocket Manual of General Thoracic Surgery*, DOI 10.1007/978-3-319-17497-6_2,
© Springer International Publishing Switzerland 2015

## Double Lumen Tube (DLT)

- DLTs are the preferred method for lung isolation.
- Benefits include selective deflation and re-inflation of either lung, the ability to suction an independent lung prior to re-inflation, and a lower risk of dislodgment compared to other modalities.
- Specific DLTs are available for the left and right main stem bronchi, and are available in different sizes (adults: 35–41 Fr; children: 28–32 Fr). Correct size selection of DLT requires careful review of CT scan or chest X-ray. The most accurate way to choose DLT size is based on the direct measurement of the left bronchial width using CT or chest X-ray if the left bronchus is seen [1]. If the left bronchus is not seen, size can be calculated using tracheal width [2]:

  - Tracheal width ≥18 mm: 41 Fr
  - Tracheal width ≥16 mm: 39 Fr
  - Tracheal width ≥15 mm: 37 Fr
  - Tracheal width ≥14 mm: 35 Fr

- For emergency cases where imaging is not readily available, the following general guidelines can also be used [3]:

  - Male >170 cm: 41 Fr
  - Male <170 cm: 39 Fr
  - Female >160 cm: 37 Fr
  - Female <160 cm: 35 Fr

## Endobronchial Intubation

- Traditional endotracheal tube or a specially designed endobronchial tube is advanced into the main stem bronchi.
- This method might be favorable in pediatric patients, or patients undergoing carinal resection.
- Endobronchial intubation with traditional endotracheal tube should only be reserved for emergency situations due to risk of inadequate single-lung ventilation and/or failure of lung isolation.

## Bronchial Blocker (BB)

- Specially designed BBs or Fogarty vascular embolectomy catheters can be used.
- In patients with impaired pulmonary function who cannot tolerate full independent lung collapse, a selective lobe blocking can be achieved with the combination of bronchial blockers and direct visualization using a pediatric bronchoscope.
- BBs are also useful in patients with tracheostomy tubes or patients with difficult airway, where a double lumen tube insertion may not be feasible.
- Dislodgment of a BB may obstruct ventilation, especially when placed on the short right main stem bronchus. This requires immediate deflation and repositioning.

# Postoperative Care

## Clinical Pathways (Tables 2.1 and 2.2)

- Fast-track and enhanced recovery pathways in thoracic surgery utilizing a written, multimodal, evidence-based, step-by-step approach to perioperative care are increasingly utilized.
- Basic principles include written daily patient education goals, smoking cessation, preoperative physiotherapy, nutrition supplementation, epidural pain control, early mobilization, early feeding, and early drain removal.

  - Implementation of these pathways has shown improvement in both hospital stay (after esophagectomy and lung resection) and postoperative complications (after lung resection) [4–6].

## Fluid Management

- Thoracic surgery does not induce large fluid shifts and intravascular fluid losses compared to other surgical procedures.

TABLE 2.1. Comparison of postoperative care milestones between traditional care and an enhanced-recovery pathway implemented at the McGill University Health Centre (Montreal, Canada) for lung resection.

| | Traditional care | Enhanced-recovery pathway |
|---|---|---|
| Patient education | Variable | Standardized preoperative education protocol |
| Drain (urine) | Variable | POD #1: removal |
| Drain (chest tube) | Variable weaning protocol | POD #0: −20 cm suction |
| | | POD #3: removal of second chest tube if <450 mL/24 h and no air leak |
| Nutrition | Surgeon discretion | POD #0: clear fluid |
| | | POD #1: diet as tolerated |
| Activity | Mobility encouraged by team | POD #0: up in chair |
| | | POD #1: ambulate in hallway BID |
| | | POD #2: ambulate >18 m TID |
| | | POD #3: ambulate >75 m TID |
| Target discharge | None | POD #4 |

TABLE 2.2. Comparison of postoperative care milestones between traditional care and an enhanced-recovery pathway implemented at the McGill University Health Centre (Montreal, Canada) for esophagectomy.

| | Traditional care | Enhanced-recovery pathway |
|---|---|---|
| Patient education | Variable | Standardized preoperative education protocol |
| Drain (urine) | Variable | POD #1 |
| Drain (chest tube) | Removal 1 day after resumption of feeds | POD #5 |
| Nutrition | Surgeon discretion | POD #3: clear fluid |
| | | POD #5: post-esophagectomy diet |
| Nasogastric tube | Removal after barium swallow (POD #7) | POD #2 |
| Contrast study | POD #7: barium swallow | None |
| Target discharge | None | POD #6 |

- Collapse and re-expansion of lung parenchyma, heterogeneous pulmonary compliance in lateral decubitus position, elevated positive pressure ventilatory pressures, or increased pulmonary arterial pressures during single-lung ventilation may induce pulmonary edema that should be monitored and managed postoperatively.
- Avoiding fluid overload through judicious, if not restricted, crystalloid and colloid administration intraoperatively and postoperatively is therefore critical in all thoracic patients, especially in patients with limited pulmonary reserve, or with cases requiring increasing pulmonary resection, where the remaining lung is subjected to the entire cardiac output. Fluid restriction while maintaining adequate end-organ perfusion is essential.
- Transient hypotension and decreased urine output may be seen due to relative rather than absolute hypovolemia in patients with high thoracic epidural analgesia and should be managed with judicious fluid administration, decreasing epidural dosing as well as its concentration of local anesthetic, and occasionally using low dose vasopressor administration.

## Analgesia

- Principles of analgesia include [7]:

  1. Multimodal analgesia (e.g., acetaminophen, NSAID and opiate)
  2. Meticulous and continuous attention to each patient's pain, while dynamically adjusting analgesia, particularly in the first 48 h
  3. Identifying patients at increased risk for postoperative pain
  4. Targeted use of epidural and intercostal blockade

- Thoracotomy incisions may be very painful (Fig. 2.1), impairing adequate mobilization, inspiration and expectoration, leading to atelectasis, retention of secretions, infection or worse. Inadequate analgesia contributes to a

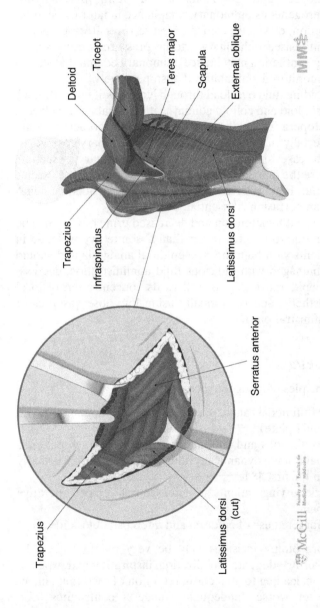

FIG. 2.1. Typical posterolateral thoracotomy incision. *Used with permission from the McGill University Health Centre Patient Education Office.*

significant number of postoperative complications in these patients. Inadequate control of pain on postoperative days 1 and 2 is an independent predictor of chronic post-thoracotomy pain. It is thus imperative to control pain effectively and immediately.

- The use of high thoracic epidural anesthesia is associated with improved pain control and decreased risk of pulmonary complications (such as pneumonia, atelectasis, prolonged mechanical ventilation, and re-intubation from respiratory failure), compared to patient-controlled analgesia and narcotic administration [8]. There is also a reduction in opioid consumption.
- Thoracoscopic incisions are generally far less painful; however, chronic pain may occur due to levering a trocar on the rib and neurovascular bundle above. Preemptive analgesia with intercostal nerve blocks and local infiltration is an essential adjunct to multimodal oral and intravenous analgesia.
- Over-sedation should be avoided when switching patients to oral or subcutaneous narcotics, as this may lead to subsequent hypoventilation and hypercarbia.
- Risk factors for poor postoperative pain control include: preoperative patient preparedness, high opioid tolerance, young age, psychological factors (e.g., preoperative anxiety, depression, neuroticism), chronic pain, incision type (thoracotomy > VATS), and rib resection [9–13].

## Chest Tube Management

- Chest tubes are routinely placed in virtually all operations whereby the parietal pleura has been entered to allow for evacuation of air, detection and management of air leaks, and drainage of hemothorax, chylothorax, enteric content, or other types of pleural effusions.
- Principles of chest tube placement include being positioned for optimal drainage (fluid: posterior and basal; air: apical and anterior), with tube caliber directed at expected

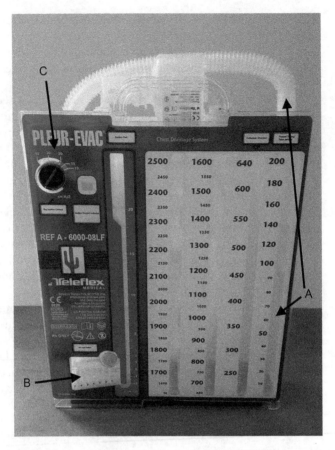

Fig. 2.2. Chest tube collection chamber unit. (**a**) Collection chamber, (**b**) water seal, (**c**) suction.

output (large-bore chest tube for sanguinous fluid; pigtail for air and serous fluid).
- Postoperatively, the patient is asked to voluntarily cough or perform a Valsalva's maneuver and the water sealed chamber is observed for bubbles (Fig. 2.2). The fluid level

in the water chamber should move up and down with deep respiration and coughing.

- Stationary fluid level in the water seal indicates either intra-thoracic or extra-thoracic tube blockage.
- Large swings in the fluid level indicate the presence of a large residual pleural space.

• Persistent air leak can be detected by suddenly placing (or increasing) the chamber on suction and observing a sudden rush of air through the system. For patients with small air leaks, the chest tube can be clamped for a couple of hours and then unclamped while on vacuum suction to observe the sudden rush of air; however, clamping overnight is neither necessary nor advisable.

**Suction:**

• Placement of chest tubes on suction rather than water seal after lung resection has not been shown to affect the duration of chest tube, duration of hospital stay, or duration of air leak. However, placing chest tube on suction is associated with a lower incidence of pneumothorax after pulmonary resection [14, 15].
• As a principle of management, the minimal suction to achieve intended pleural drainage objectives is optimal.
• Chest tube placed in post-pneumonectomy patients should not be on suction due to the risk of mediastinal shift and cardiac herniation.

**Removal:**

• The ideal volume drainage to predict safe removal of chest tubes is unknown. 200 mL/24 h with no air leak is commonly quoted as the threshold for removal; however, there is no evidence to support this.

- Chest tubes can be safely removed with drainage volumes of up to 500 mL/24 h without increasing the risk of fluid re-accumulation [16, 17].
- Commonly, the target removal date of the second tube after a lobectomy is on day 3 if there is <300 mL of non-chylous fluid in 24 h with no air leak.
- Chest tubes should be removed sequentially and each tube should be removed while off suction, with simultaneous application of an occlusive dressing to prevent air entry during its removal.

## Respiratory Care

- It is imperative for patients to maintain the ability to deliver an effective cough (pulmonary toilet) and to maintain good bronchial hygiene.
- Incisional pain can lead to significant chest wall splinting, preventing proper airway clearance of secretions and mucus plugs. This is further exacerbated by a strong smoking history and chronic bronchitis.

  – Placing a pillow over the incision while coughing reduces pain.

- Early ambulation, fluid restriction, aggressive pain control, chest physiotherapy, and prevention of over-sedation with narcotic medications all contribute to a better pulmonary recovery in the postoperative period.
- Nasotracheal suctioning, flexible bronchoscopy, mechanical ventilation may be required, especially in patients with poor preoperative pulmonary function.
- Other supportive therapies include (as necessary):

  – Humidified oxygen
  – Bronchodilators
  – N-acetylcysteine
  – Diuretics
  – High flow, high humidity oxygen

# Postoperative Complications

- The Thoracic Morbidity and Mortality (TM&M) classification is a system to standardize and grade the presence and severity of surgical complications after non-cardiac thoracic surgery (available at: http://www.ottawatmm.org[18])

## Cardiac Complications

- Thoracic surgery patients are at high-risk of cardiac complications due to similar risk factors (e.g., smoking).
- The most common are myocardial ischemia, arrhythmias and heart failure.
- All patients should undergo thorough preoperative screening for cardiac comorbidities.

**Atrial Fibrillation:**

- 15–40 % of all patients undergoing major thoracic surgery will develop atrial fibrillation depending on preoperative left-atrial function [19].
- Management should address rate-control, with anticoagulation indicated after several days of refractory fibrillation, along with treatment of any precipitating factors (e.g., electrolyte imbalance — potassium and magnesium, pain, sepsis, hypoxemia, hemothorax).

## Respiratory Complications

- Most common complication after thoracic surgery.
- Workup of patients in respiratory distress includes: chest X-ray, ECG, lab-work (CBC, serum chemistries, renal function tests, arterial blood gas, cardiac enzymes) and additional studies as necessary.

**Respiratory Failure**

- Can occur secondary to multiple causes, including pneumonia, pulmonary edema, acute respiratory distress

syndrome (ARDS), aspiration, mucus plug, atelectasis, heart failure, hypoventilation, sepsis, and pulmonary embolus.
- Management should address the suspected cause(s), while providing adequate oxygenation and/or ventilatory support as required. Flexible bronchoscopy can also be done for pulmonary toilet and mucus plugs.

**Aspiration (Fig. 2.3)**

- Most common in patients after esophagectomy secondary to vagotomy and subsequent dysmotility.
- Early mobilization and ambulation promotes better pulmonary function and decreases incidence of aspiration.

**Pulmonary Edema (Fig. 2.4)**

- Can be caused by pulmonary hypertension (increased resistance after lung resection) and impaired lymphatic drainage after lymph node dissection, favoring fluid accumulation and edema.
- *Post-pneumonectomy Syndrome:*
  - Severe pulmonary edema occurring early after pneumonectomy, characterized by diffuse infiltrates, significant right-to-left shunting, and hypoxemia.
  - Presentation and management is similar to acute lung injury or ARDS—namely, minimizing lung injury (including lung-protective ventilation and avoiding over resuscitation).

**Prolonged Air Leaks**

- Persistent air leak >5 days, frequently occur after lung resection (15 %)
- Increases length of stay and readmissions, with substantial economic burden
- Strategies to decrease incidence of air leaks:
  - Sealants: shown to reduce postoperative air leaks and time to chest tube removal, however not always associated with reduced hospital length-of-stay [20].

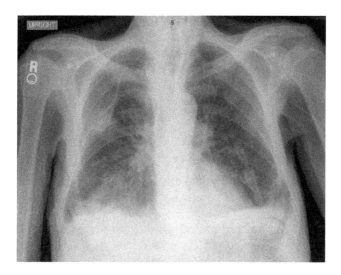

FIG. 2.3. Chest X-ray of a patient who experienced aspiration following lung resection. A consolidation is seen in the right lower lobe.

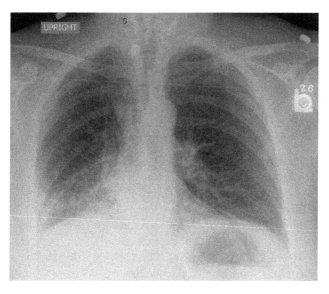

FIG. 2.4. Chest X-ray of a patient with pulmonary edema who required diuresis postoperatively.

Routine use unlikely to be cost-effective
Should be considered in high-risk patients (e.g., bullec-
    tomy, severe emphysema)

- Flap coverage
- Tenting of the lung
- Use of Bovine patch to buttress staple in high-risk
  patients

**Bronchopleural Fistula (BPF)**

- Breakdown of the stump can occur secondary to ischemia,
  tumor recurrence, poor wound healing or empyema resulting in BPF.
- BPFs can be hard to distinguish from persistent air leaks,
  but should be suspected in moderate to severe air leaks,
  especially in immunocompromised patients.
- Diagnosis is confirmed by flexible bronchoscopy.
- Hemodynamically stable patients can be initially managed
  conservatively by tube thoracostomy, antibiotics, and
  respiratory support (+/− mechanical ventilation).

  - If ventilatory support is required, airflow through the
    leaking stump should be minimized. This can be done
    using lung-isolation techniques.

- Failure of conservative management mandates surgical
  reinforcement of the stump with a muscle flap.

**Deep Vein Thrombosis (DVT) and Pulmonary Embolism**

- Thoracic patients with malignancies are at high risk for
  developing DVTs and pulmonary embolisms, and should
  be maintained on prophylactic anticoagulation throughout
  admission.
- With sequential compression devices used intraoperatively, along with postoperative prophylactic
  anticoagulation, rates of clinically significant venous
  thrombosis are expected to be low (<2 %).

**Thoracic Duct Injury**

- Patients undergoing extensive mediastinal dissection such as during esophagectomy are prone to duct injuries.

    - Incidence: 1–3 % post-esophagectomy [21].

- Diagnosis is usually made after initiation of enteral feeding which causes an accumulation of a triglyceride-rich milky fluid in the chest cavity. *See Chapter 4: Pleural Disorders (Chylothorax)*
- Treatment of low output leaks (<1 L/day) can be done conservatively, by keeping the chest tube drainage under water seal and off vacuum suction.
- High output thoracic duct injuries (>1 L/day) usually require surgical ligation.
- Recent randomized controlled trial suggests that mass ligation decreases the risk of chylothorax [21].

**Vocal Cord Paralysis**

- Recurrent laryngeal nerve injury can occur during esophagectomy, cervical mediastinoscopy, and mediastinal lymph node dissection.
- Injury may lead anywhere from weak voice, hoarseness, and ineffective cough, to permanent voice loss, stridor, and acute airway obstruction.
- Vocal cords are best assessed by visualization using a fiber-optic laryngoscope.
- Higher rates of recurrent nerve trauma after cervical anastomosis for esophagectomy compared to thoracic anastomosis (OR 7.14, 95 % CI 1.09–10.78) [22]

## *Esophageal Complications*

**Esophageal Anastomotic Leak**

- Most leaks occur either early <48 h or after 1 week, secondary to conduit ischemia and necrosis or staple line dehiscence.

- Early anastomotic leak (<48 h) reflects a technical complication or conduit necrosis.
- Delayed anastomotic leak (7–10 days) reflects ischemia of the conduit.

• Cervical anastomosis

- Higher leak rate: 10–25 % (OR 4.73, 95 % CI 1.61-13.9) [23–25]
- Lower mortality

• Intrathoracic anastomosis

- Lower leak rate: 3–12 % [23–25]
- Higher mortality

• Risk factors include: cardiovascular disease (heart failure, coronary artery disease, peripheral vascular disease), smoking, use of vasopressors, location (higher risk in cervical), poor nutritional status and tension on the anastomosis [24].
• Technical factors affecting anastomotic integrity—no difference in [25]:

- Hand-sewn vs. stapled
- Minimally invasive vs. open
- Anterior vs. posterior route of reconstruction
- Ischemic conditioning of gastric conduit

• Leaks associated with reduced long-term survival after esophagectomy [26]

Diagnosis

• Early leaks should be suspected with increase in chest tube drainage volume, drainage of enteric/bilious content, drainage of coffee ground fluid from the nasogastric tube, in addition to fever, leukocytosis, subcutaneous emphysema and signs of sepsis from mediastinitis and empyema.
• Late anastomotic leaks present more subtly and might require esophagogastroscopy to evaluate the extent of the leak and graft ischemia.

- Diagnosis can be confirmed by CT (with oral contrast), contrast esophagogram or esophagogastroscopy (to look for extent of leak and viability of the conduit)

  – Many centers advocate for routine contrast esophagogram prior to feeding; however, this is not a universal practice and highly controversial.
  – Many institutions perform contrast esophagogram only based on clinical suspicion, due to its low sensitivity, high false-negative rate and limited impact on patient management [27, 28].

Management

- *All patients*: antibiotics, controlled drainage (chest tube), nutritional support (enteric), and aggressive resuscitation.
- *Early fulminant leak (<48 h)*: re-exploration, debridement, and revision of anastomosis.

  – Either primarily repaired, reinforced (with serratus, omentum, pericardium, or stent), or diverted with delayed reconstruction (esophagostomy spit fistula, gastrostomy, feeding jejunostomy, and colon interposition at 3–6 months) depending on time to management and degree of contamination.

- *Cervical anastomosis (2–10 days):* leaks can be managed by opening the skin incision (to allow for drainage and assessment of gastric viability) and packing the wound.
- *Intrathoracic anastomosis (2–10 days):*

  – Higher mortality rate compared to cervical anastomosis
  – Small leaks in stable patients can be managed conservatively with or without stenting for partial tissue loss
  – Large and uncontrolled leaks and conduit necrosis require re-exploration and debridement.

    Either primarily repaired, reinforced (with serratus, omentum, pericardium or stent), or diverted with delayed reconstruction (esophagostomy spit fistula, gastrostomy, feeding jejunostomy, and colon interposition at 3–6 months) depending on time to management and degree of contamination.

- Smaller leaks that are managed conservatively can develop strictures requiring future dilation.

**Delayed Gastric Emptying**

- Occurs after significant manipulation, resection of the stomach and transaction of the vagus nerve.
- Clinical presentation: regurgitation/vomiting, aspiration, acid reflux, early satiety
- Barium swallow to confirm diagnosis
- Prevention:
  - Narrow conduit
  - Avoidance of conduit redundancy or twisting
  - Adequate closure of hiatus

# References

1. Brodsky JB, Lemmens HJ. Tracheal width and left double-lumen tube size: a formula to estimate left-bronchial width. J Clin Anesth. 2005;17(4):267–70.
2. Brodsky JB, Macario A, Mark JB. Tracheal diameter predicts double-lumen tube size: a method for selecting left double-lumen tubes. Anesth Analg. 1996;82(4):861–4.
3. Orlewicz MS, Coleman AE, Choromanski D, Meyers AD. Double-Lumen endotracheal tube placement. Medscape. http://emedicine.medscape.com/article/1999993-overview. Accessed 26 Jan 26 2015.
4. Li C et al. An enhanced recovery pathway decreases duration of stay after esophagectomy. Surgery. 2012;152(4):606–14. discussion 614-6.
5. Numan RC et al. A clinical audit in a multidisciplinary care path for thoracic surgery: an instrument for continuous quality improvement. Lung Cancer. 2012;78(3):270–5.
6. Muhling B, Orend KH, Sunder-Plassmann L. Fast track in thoracic surgery. Chirurg. 2009;80(8):706–10.

7. Bottiger BA, Esper SA, Stafford-Smith M. Pain management strategies for thoracotomy and thoracic pain syndromes. Semin Cardiothorac Vasc Anesth. 2014;18(1):45–56.

8. Popping DM et al. Protective effects of epidural analgesia on pulmonary complications after abdominal and thoracic surgery: a meta-analysis. Arch Surg. 2008;143(10):990–9. discussion 1000.

9. Ip HY et al. Predictors of postoperative pain and analgesic consumption: a qualitative systematic review. Anesthesiology. 2009; 111(3):657–77.

10. Bachiocco V et al. Intensity, latency and duration of postthoracotomy pain: relationship to personality traits. Funct Neurol. 1990;5(4):321–32.

11. Caumo W et al. Preoperative predictors of moderate to intense acute postoperative pain in patients undergoing abdominal surgery. Acta Anaesthesiol Scand. 2002;46(10):1265–71.

12. Landreneau RJ et al. Postoperative pain-related morbidity: video-assisted thoracic surgery versus thoracotomy. Ann Thorac Surg. 1993;56(6):1285–9.

13. Egbert LD et al. Reduction of postoperative pain by encouragement and instruction of patients. A study of doctor–patient rapport. N Engl J Med. 1964;270:825–7.

14. Coughlin SM, Emmerton-Coughlin HM, Malthaner R. Management of chest tubes after pulmonary resection: a systematic review and meta-analysis. Can J Surg. 2012;55(4): 264–70.

15. Cerfolio RJ, Bass C, Katholi CR. Prospective randomized trial compares suction versus water seal for air leaks. Ann Thorac Surg. 2001;71(5):1613–7.

16. Cerfolio RJ, Bryant AS. Results of a prospective algorithm to remove chest tubes after pulmonary resection with high output. J Thorac Cardiovasc Surg. 2008;135(2):269–73.

17. Bjerregaard LS et al. Early chest tube removal after video-assisted thoracic surgery lobectomy with serous fluid production up to 500 ml/day. Eur J Cardiothorac Surg. 2014;45(2):241–6.

18. Seely AJ et al. Systematic classification of morbidity and mortality after thoracic surgery. Ann Thorac Surg. 2010;90(3):936–42. discussion 942.

19. Raman T et al. Preoperative left atrial dysfunction and risk of postoperative atrial fibrillation complicating thoracic surgery. J Thorac Cardiovasc Surg. 2012;143(2):482–7.

20. Belda-Sanchis J et al. Surgical sealant for preventing air leaks after pulmonary resections in patients with lung cancer. Cochrane Database Syst Rev. 2010;1, CD003051.

21. Lai FC et al. Prevention of chylothorax complicating extensive esophageal resection by mass ligation of thoracic duct: a random control study. Ann Thorac Surg. 2011;91(6):1770–4.
22. Biere SS et al. Cervical or thoracic anastomosis after esophagectomy for cancer: a systematic review and meta-analysis. Dig Surg. 2011;28(1):29–35.
23. Martin LW et al. Management of intrathoracic leaks following esophagectomy. Adv Surg. 2006;40:173–90.
24. Kassis ES et al. Predictors of anastomotic leak after esophagectomy: an analysis of the society of thoracic surgeons general thoracic database. Ann Thorac Surg. 2013;96(6):1919–26.
25. Markar SR et al. Technical factors that affect anastomotic integrity following esophagectomy: systematic review and meta-analysis. Ann Surg Oncol. 2013;20(13):4274–81.
26. Kofoed SC et al. Intrathoracic anastomotic leakage after gastro-esophageal cancer resection is associated with reduced long-term survival. World J Surg. 2014;38(1):114–9.
27. Solomon DG, Sasaki CT, Salem RR. An evaluation of the routine use of contrast radiography as a screening test for cervical anastomotic integrity after esophagectomy. Am J Surg. 2012; 203(4):467–71.
28. Tirnaksiz MB et al. Effectiveness of screening aqueous contrast swallow in detecting clinically significant anastomotic leaks after esophagectomy. Eur Surg Res. 2005;37(2):123–8.

# Chapter 3
# Lung and Airway Disorders

**Monisha Sudarshan, Hussam Alamri,**
**and Mohammed Al-Mahroos**

## Section 1: Lung Cancer
*Primary Lung Cancer*

### Epidemiology [1, 2]

- Second most commonly diagnosed cancer—accounts for 14 % of new cancer cases in the USA
- Leading cause of cancer death (27 % of all cancer deaths) in the USA
- Estimated 25,500 and 201,144 new lung cancer diagnoses among Canadians and Americans, respectively
- Incidence decreasing amongst men, and stabilising amongst women
- Overall 5-year survival of 15 % (in early stage disease, 5-year survival: 60–70 %)

M. Sudarshan, M.D., M.P.H. (✉)
Department of Surgery, McGill University Health Center,
1650 Cedar Avenue, Montreal, QC, Canada H3G 1A4
e-mail: monisha.sudarshan@mail.mcgill.ca

H. Alamri, M.D. • M. Al-Mahroos, M.D.
Department of Surgery, McGill University Health Center,
Montreal, QC, Canada

A. Madani et al. (eds.), *Pocket Manual of General Thoracic Surgery*, DOI 10.1007/978-3-319-17497-6_3,
© Springer International Publishing Switzerland 2015

35

**Risk Factors**

- Cigarette smoking: attributable for up to 80 % of lung cancers; 15 % of heavy smokers develop cancer

  - Increased duration contributes more risk than daily usage [3]

- Other: Asbestos, Arsenic, Chromium, Nickel exposure, organic chemical, radon, iatrogenic radiation exposure

**Pathology**

- *Non-Small-Cell Lung Carcinomas (NSCLC)*

  - *Adenocarcinoma*

    Most common histology (40 %)
    Originates from mucin-producing cells of bronchial epithelium
    Mostly located peripherally (outer third of lung)
    *Bronchoalveolar carcinoma:* variant of adenocarcinoma with the best overall prognosis

    - Highly differentiated, spreads along alveolar walls with non-destructive *lepidic* growth; can present as slowly growing solid component of a ground glass opacity (GGO), a diffuse parenchymal infiltrate, multiple nodules or a solitary nodule

  - *Squamous Cell Carcinoma*

    25 % of lung cancers
    Mostly located centrally with spread along bronchus resulting in extrinsic compression
    Characteristic central necrosis and cavitation (10 %)

  - *Large cell undifferentiated carcinoma*

    Mostly located peripherally

- *Small-Cell Lung Carcinomas (SCLC)*

  - 20 % of all lung cancers
  - Centrally located (inner two thirds of lung)

- Strong association with smoking [4]
- Early and aggressive mediastinal lymph nodes and distal metastases

- *Carcinoids*

  - Neuroendocrine tumours of the lung occur as a spectrum based on aggressiveness:

  Kulchitsky I: well-differentiated typical carcinoids

  - Typically centrally located in bronchi

  Kulchitsky II: atypical carcinoids (less differentiated than typical carcinoids)
  Kulchitsky III: poorly differentiated SCLC

  - Typical and atypical carcinoids consist of 5 % of all lung cancers.
  - Both lymphatogenous and systemic metastases are rare with typical carcinoids.

## Clinical Presentation

- *Asymptomatic*: Patients typically present with an incidental finding of an abnormal chest radiograph during an unrelated medical visit.
- *Bronchoplumonary*: cough (new, or change from previously stable), increased sputum production, change in level of dyspnea with exertion, wheezing, haemoptysis, fever (post-obstructive pneumonia)
- *Regional Extra-pulmonary from Invasion:*

  - Chest wall and pleura: chest pain, malignant pleural effusion
  - Recurrent laryngeal nerve: hoarseness, ineffective cough, permanent voice loss, stridor, acute airway obstruction
  - Superior vena cava (SVC): SVC syndrome (facial and upper-extremity edema)
  - Cervical sympathetic ganglia: Horner syndrome (miosis, ptosis, anhidrosis)

- Brachial Plexus: pancoast syndrome (shoulder/arm pain and hand muscle weakness/atrophy
- Phrenic nerve paralysis: hypoventilation
- Oesophagus: dysphagia, bronchoesophageal fistula

- *Distant Metastasis*: most common sites include bone, liver, adrenal glands, brain and lung (contralateral side)

  - Signs and symptoms related to end-organ involvement
  - Constitutional symptoms: anorexia, malaise, weight loss, fatigue

- *Paraneoplastic Syndromes*:

  - Occur in 10 % of patients; more common with SCLC.
  - Includes: metabolic (Cushing's, carcinoid syndrome, hypercalcemia, syndrome of inappropriate antidiuretic hormone), skeletal (clubbing, hypertrophic pulmonary osteoarthropathy), neuromuscular (polymyositis, Eaton–Lambert, peripheral neuropathy), dermatologic (acanthosis nigricans) and vascular (thrombophlebitis) syndromes.

**Workup and Staging (Table 3.1)**

- Laboratory tests (CBC, serum chemistries, renal function tests, LDH, liver function tests)
- Pulmonary Function Tests (PFTs)

  - *See* Chap. 1*: Preoperative Evaluation of the Thoracic Patient.*

- Radiographic Evaluation

  - *Chest X-Ray*

    First-line modality, usually followed by CT for detailed evaluation.

    Lesions at a minimum of 7–10 mm in diameter can be visualised.

    Assess for number and sites of lesion (central/peripheral), secondary effects of tumour (consolidation/atelectasis due to segmental or lobar collapse), presence of effusion, and advanced bone lesions.

TABLE 3.1 TNM staging classification for lung cancer.

Lung cancer TNM staging

*Primary tumour (T)*

| | |
|---|---|
| T1 | Tumour ≤3 cm diameter, surrounded by lung or visceral pleura, without invasion more proximal than lobar bronchus |
| T1a | Tumour ≤2 cm in diameter |
| T1b | Tumour >2 cm but ≤3 cm in diameter |
| T2 | Tumour >3 cm but ≤7 cm, or tumour with any of the following features: |
| | – Involves main bronchus, ≥2 cm distal to carina |
| | – Invades visceral pleura |
| | – Associated with atelectasis or obstructive pneumonitis that extends to the hilar region but does not involve the entire lung |
| T2a | Tumour >3 cm but ≤5 cm |
| T2b | Tumour >5 cm but ≤7 cm |
| T3 | Tumour >7 cm or any of the following: |
| | – Directly invades any of the following: chest wall, diaphragm, phrenic nerve, mediastinal pleura, parietal pericardium, main bronchus <2 cm from carina (without involvement of carina) |
| | – Atelectasis or obstructive pneumonitis of the entire lung |
| | – Separate tumour nodules in the same lobe |
| T4 | Tumour of any size that invades the mediastinum, heart, great vessels, trachea, recurrent laryngeal nerve, oesophagus, vertebral body, carina, or with separate tumour nodules in a different ipsilateral lobe |

*Regional lymph nodes (N)*

| | |
|---|---|
| N0 | No regional lymph node metastases |
| N1 | Metastasis in ipsilateral peribronchial and/or ipsilateral hilar lymph nodes and intrapulmonary nodes, including involvement by direct extension |
| N2 | Metastasis in ipsilateral mediastinal and/or subcarinal lymph node(s) |
| N3 | Metastasis in contralateral mediastinal, contralateral hilar, ipsilateral or contralateral scalene, or supraclavicular lymph node(s) |

(continued)

Table 3.1 (continued)

*Distant metastasis (M)*

| | |
|---|---|
| M0 | No distant metastasis |
| M1 | Distant metastasis |
| M1a | Separate tumour nodule(s) in a contralateral lobe; tumour with pleural nodules or malignant pleural or pericardial effusion |
| M1b | Distant metastasis (in extra-thoracic organs) |

| Stage | T | N | M |
|---|---|---|---|
| IA | T1a, T1b | N0 | M0 |
| IB | T2a | N0 | M0 |
| IIA | T1,T2a | N1 | M0 |
| | T2b | N0 | M0 |
| IIB | T2b | N1 | M0 |
| | T3 | N0 | M0 |
| IIIA | T1, T2 | N2 | M0 |
| | T3 | N1,N2 | M0 |
| | T4 | N0,N1 | M0 |
| IIIB | T4 | N2 | M0 |
| | Any T | N3 | M0 |
| IV | Any T | Any N | M1 |

*Used with permission of the American Joint Committee on Cancer (AJCC), Chicago, IL.* The original and primary source for this information is the AJCC Cancer Staging Manual, Seventh Edition (2010) published by Springer Science + Business Media

– *CT Chest* (with IV contrast)

Used to evaluate size, location, number of lung lesions, features of malignancy (scalloped borders, spiculations, corona radiata, lack of calcifications, ground glass opacities [5]), tumour cavitation and necrosis, secondary effects (including atelectasis, post-obstructive pneumonia, pleural effusion), extent of invasion into adjacent structures, chest wall or mediastinum, and mediastinal lymphadenopathy.

Lymph node metastasis sensitivity: 51 %; specificity: 86 % [6]

- Lymph nodes between 10 and 15 mm have a 50 % risk of malignant involvement, while those >15 mm have a 67 % risk.

Abdominal cuts also included to look for distant metastases (e.g. adrenals and liver).

Brain CT (with IV contrast) should be performed if MRI is not available to rule out metastases in selected patients.

– *PET-CT*

Helps to identify diseased nodes in normal sized lymph nodes on CT [7], distinguish benign and malignant pulmonary nodules and other sites with remote metastasis.

- Minimal role in patients with obvious metastatic disease.

A systematic review on the diagnostic properties of PET-CT for mediastinal lymph node metastasis demonstrated a sensitivity 83 %, specificity 96 %, and accuracy >90 % [6, 8].

Although it has high sensitivity (96 %) for discrimination of malignant from benign nodules, it has lower specificity (78 %) and a positive-predictive value of 91 % due to false positives secondary to increased uptake in inflammatory, granulomatous, or infectious conditions [8, 9].

Some tumours (i.e. typical carcinoids) tend to have low metabolic activity and are not be PET-avid.

If any uncertainty exists, confirmation of positive findings should be made with tissue diagnosis before ruling out pulmonary resection for lung cancer.

– *MRI*

Used for tumour delineation with suspected local invasion into brachial plexus, superior sulcus vessels, vertebral body or spinal cord, and for brain metastases. Otherwise it does not offer significant advantages over CT.

MRI is the gold standard for evaluating the brain for any evidence of metastases in selected patients.

- Invasive Staging (Non-Surgical Tissue Diagnosis):

  - *Percutaneous transthoracic needle aspiration (TTNA)*

    For peripherally located lesions >1 cm (lacks accuracy for subcentimetric lesions)

    TTNA allows the clinician to secure a tissue diagnosis preoperatively, thereby avoiding potentially unnecessary pulmonary resection if a benign diagnosis is made (e.g. necrotizing granuloma).

    For new, growing and resectable nodules, TTNA may not change management.

    Carries risk of pneumothorax (10–30 %), pulmonary haemorrhage (5–20 %), transient haemoptysis (2 %) and rarely, air embolism (<0.1 %) [10, 11].

  - *Flexible bronchoscopy* (Fig. 3.1)

    Includes forceps biopsy, brushings, saline lavage, transbronchial needle aspiration (TBNA).

    Can be used to sample centrally located primary tumours and lymph nodes.

    Adjunct guidance improved with fluoroscopy for TBNA.

  - *Endobronchial ultrasound (EBUS) guided TBNA*

    Especially useful for paratracheal, subcarinal or hilar lymph nodes.

    Cannot sample subaortic or paraesophageal lymph nodes.

    Can sample primary tumour (superior to bronchoscopy for masses <3 cm [12]).

    95 % Sensitivity, 100 % specificity in several studies [13, 14].

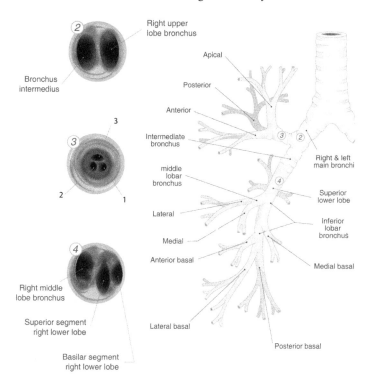

FIG. 3.1. Tracheobronchial tree with intra-luminal bronchoscopic view. *Used with permission from the McGill University Health Centre Patient Education Office.*

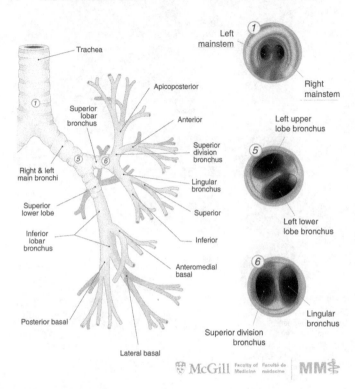

Fɪɢ. 3.1. (continued)

- *Transesophageal endoscopic ultrasound guided FNA (EUS-FNA)*

   Especially useful for subcarinal, aortopulmonary, paraesophageal and pulmonary ligament lymph nodes. Sensitivity: 92 %; specificity: 100 %; accuracy: 97 % [15].

   Used in conjunction with EBUS to sample all lymph node stations.

   • EBUS-FNA: anterior and superior lymph nodes
   • EUS-FNA: posterior and inferior lymph nodes

   Can also be used to characterise the primary tumour's extent of invasion.

- Invasive Staging (Surgical Tissue Diagnosis):

  – *Cervical mediastinoscopy*

    Can be done using direct optic visualisation or video-assisted mediastinoscopy with sensitivity and specificity of 78 % and 100 % respectively, and 11 % false-negative rate [16].

    Samples upper and lower paratracheal lymph nodes above the aortic arch.

    Access to anterior subcarinal and bilateral hilar nodes are technically challenging.

    Not a necessary or routine step in staging (can be eliminated in clinical T1aN0 disease—namely, tumours that are <2 cm in maximal diameter, with negative PET-CT).

  – *Chamberlain's procedure (anterior mediastinotomy)*

    Access through the second or third intercostal space to left paratracheal, para-aortic, subaortic and subcarinal nodes.

  – *Video-Assisted Thoracic Surgery (VATS)*

    Can provide biopsies of paratracheal, azygos, paraesophageal, pulmonary ligament, subaortic and para-aortic lymph nodes.

    Patients with solitary pulmonary nodules with high suspicion for malignancy (based on nodule size, interval growth rate, and patient risk factors such as smoking history, age >40 and family history [17, 18]) can also undergo tissue diagnosis intra-operatively.

**Management—Non-Small Cell Lung Carcinoma [19]:**

- Locoregional Disease (Fig. 3.2):

  – Surgical resection is standard-of-care for localised disease.

  – Most patients with stage I disease following an R0 resection do not require adjuvant chemotherapy.

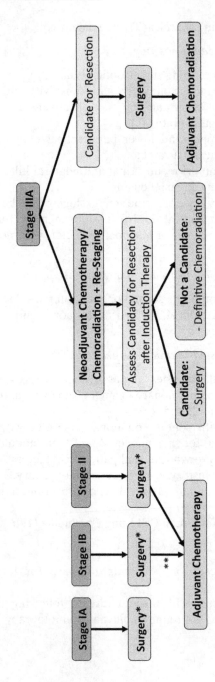

Fig. 3.2. Management algorithm for locoregional and locally advanced non-small-cell lung cancer. *: R1 resections should undergo either re-resection (with or without chemotherapy) or chemoradiation. **: High-risk features for stage IB NSCLC (e.g >4 cm) should be considered for adjuvant chemotherapy.

Meta-analysis of cisplatin-based chemotherapy in patients with resected stage 1 NSCLC showed no survival advantage (stage 1A: HR 1.40, 95%CI 0.95–2.06; stage 1B: HR 0.93, 95%CI 0.78–1.10) [20–22].

However, CALGB-9633 study suggested that adjuvant chemotherapy has a significant survival advantage in stage IB patients with tumour size >4 cm (HR 0.69, 95%CI 0.48–0.99) [23].

- Several meta-analysis and randomised controlled trials suggest a significant survival advantage for stage II patients receiving adjuvant chemotherapy (HR 0.83, 95%CI 0.73–0.95) [20, 21, 24].
- Adjuvant radiation therapy does not improve outcomes of patients with stage I disease following an R0 resection [25].

• Locally Advanced Disease (Fig. 3.2):

- Although induction therapy for stage III disease improves survival, the choice of subsequent locoregional treatment is debated.
- Neoadjuvant chemoradiation compared to neoadjuvant chemotherapy increases the pathological response rate (60–65 % vs. 20–35 %) and mediastinal node downstaging (46 % vs. 29 %, $p = 0.02$) [26, 27]. However there is no difference in progression-free survival or overall survival.
- Stage IIIA Disease (T3N1, T4N0-1):

Complex cases should undergo discussion at pulmonary oncology multidisciplinary rounds.

Patients should be assessed for resectability and the probability of achieving an R0 resection.

If unresectable, concurrent chemoradiation is the standard of treatment.

If deemed resectable, options include upfront resection followed by chemoradiation; or preoperative chemoradiation followed by surgery, with or without re-staging of the mediastinum, followed by adjuvant chemotherapy.

Certain lesions that are invading adjacent structures may benefit from aggressive en-bloc resections (including the vertebrae, carina, atrium and chest wall).

Patients with an R1 resection or unresectable disease should undergo chemoradiation.

– Stage IIIA Disease with N2 (T1-3):

Complex cases should undergo discussion at pulmonary oncology multidisciplinary rounds.

Management of locally advanced N2 disease remains controversial [28]. However it seems that tri-modality therapy (induction chemoradiation followed by surgery) compared to definitive chemoradiation without surgery, improves progression-free survival but not overall survival, except for the subset of patients undergoing lobectomy, and not pneumonectomy [29].

Definite or induction chemoradiation followed by reassessment for disease progression can guide surgical management. If there is no progression, surgery followed by adjuvant chemotherapy is an option. If there is disease progression, chemoradiation or chemotherapy for local or systemic control should be considered.

– Re-staging following induction therapy using repeat mediastinoscopy has the lowest false-negative and false-positive rates [30, 31].

• Advanced Disease (Stage IIIB and IV):

– Chemoradiation offers a survival advantage
– Palliative care to control morbidity from advanced disease (i.e. pleurodesis or long-term catheter drainage of malignant effusions, transbronchial stenting)
– Targeted systemic therapy for distant metastases

• Surgical Principles (Fig. 3.3):

– Anatomic resection in order to remove cancer and adjacent lymph nodes: lobectomy (most common),

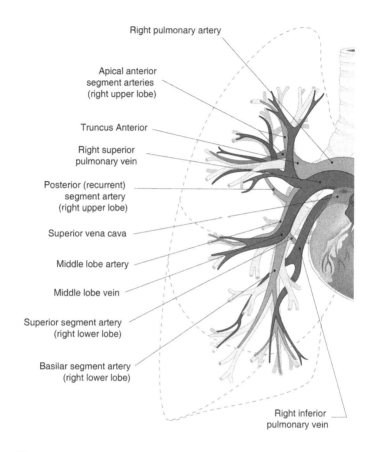

Right pulmonary artery

Apical anterior
segment arteries
(right upper lobe)

Truncus Anterior

Right superior
pulmonary vein

Posterior (recurrent)
segment artery
(right upper lobe)

Superior vena cava

Middle lobe artery

Middle lobe vein

Superior segment artery
(right lower lobe)

Basilar segment artery
(right lower lobe)

Right inferior
pulmonary vein

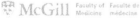
McGill   Faculty of   Faculte de
Medicine   médecine

FIG. 3.3. Pulmonary arteries and veins. *Used with permission from the McGill University Health Centre Patient Education Office.*

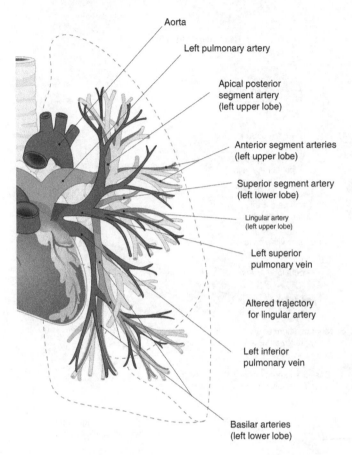

Aorta

Left pulmonary artery

Apical posterior
segment artery
(left upper lobe)

Anterior segment arteries
(left upper lobe)

Superior segment artery
(left lower lobe)

Lingular artery
(left upper lobe)

Left superior
pulmonary vein

Altered trajectory
for lingular artery

Left inferior
pulmonary vein

Basilar arteries
(left lower lobe)

FIG. 3.3.  (continued)

pneumonectomy, bilobectomy, sleeve lobectomy or segmentectomy. Lobectomy is considered standard-of-care
for stage I NSCLC in patients with adequate pulmonary
reserve.
– Non-anatomic resection (if risk of lymph node involvement is exceptionally low): wedge resection.

Lesser resections and sublobar resections are associated with higher local recurrence compared to lobectomy for stage I NSCLC [32, 33], and are reserved for select patients with small peripheral cancers (e.g. <2 cm), and/or patients with limited pulmonary reserve.

– Minimally invasive approach (VATS):

VATS lobectomy shown to decrease blood loss, chest tube drainage time, hospital length-of-stay, post-operative pain, and perioperative complications, while achieving improved oncologic outcomes compared an open approach (5-year survival rate OR 1.82, 95%CI 1.43–2.31) [34].

Relative contraindications: significant mediastinal lymphadenopathy, tumours >5 cm and centrally located tumours.

Never a contraindication for initiating an elective pulmonary oncologic resection thoracoscopically.

– Extent of lymph node dissection should include both N1 and N2 stations (minimum of 3 N2 stations).

– Sampling multi-station lymph nodes is essential for accurate staging, to allow patients to benefit from adjuvant therapy (Fig. 3.4). Although resection of lymph nodes has never been proven superior to sampling, it is good surgical practice to resect lymph nodes when possible, without incurring increased risk of harm to the patient from over-zealous and unnecessary lymph node dissection.

– Medically unfit patients should be considered for lesser resection (segmentectomy or non-anatomic wedge resection), definitive radiotherapy, chemoradiation or stereotactic radiation therapy.

• Pathologic Evaluation

– Prognostic and Predictive Biomarkers:

Epidermal growth factor receptor (EGFR) — predictive of response to EGFR-TKI therapy

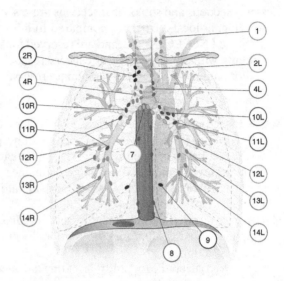

FIG. 3.4. Lymph node classification map [35]. *Used with permission from the McGill University Health Centre Patient Education Office.*

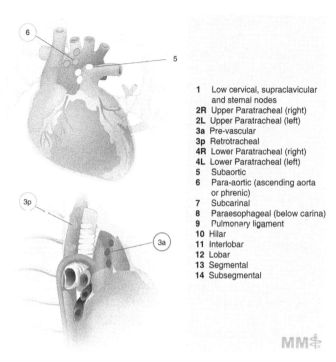

| | |
|---|---|
| **1** | Low cervical, supraclavicular and sternal nodes |
| **2R** | Upper Paratracheal (right) |
| **2L** | Upper Paratracheal (left) |
| **3a** | Pre-vascular |
| **3p** | Retrotracheal |
| **4R** | Lower Paratracheal (right) |
| **4L** | Lower Paratracheal (left) |
| **5** | Subaortic |
| **6** | Para-aortic (ascending aorta or phrenic) |
| **7** | Subcarinal |
| **8** | Paraesophageal (below carina) |
| **9** | Pulmonary ligament |
| **10** | Hilar |
| **11** | Interlobar |
| **12** | Lobar |
| **13** | Segmental |
| **14** | Subsegmental |

FIG. 3.4. (continued)

ERCC1 (improved survival and poor response to platinum chemotherapy)

KRAS oncogene (decreased survival and resistance to TKI therapy)

Anaplastic lymphoma kinase (ALK) fusion oncogene (prognostic of resistance to EGFR TKI therapy)

- Recurrence
  - Locoregional Recurrence:

    Endobronchial obstruction: radiation therapy, photodynamic therapy, laser, stents, surgery

    Resectable lung recurrence: surgery, radiation therapy

    Mediastinal lymph node recurrence: chemoradiation, systemic chemotherapy

SVC obstruction: chemoradiation, radiation therapy, SVC stent

Severe haemoptysis: radiation therapy, brachytherapy, laser, photodynamic therapy, angioembolization, surgery (endobronchial, VATS or open). *See* Chap. 3: *Lung and Airways (Haemoptysis)*.

– Distant Metastases

Diffuse brain metastases: palliative radiation therapy

Bone metastases: palliative radiation therapy, stabilisation (if at risk of fracture), bisphosphonate therapy

Disseminated metastases—testing for EGFR, ALK with subsequent targeted therapy

**Management—Small Cell Lung Carcinoma (Fig. 3.5)**

- \>50 % of patients present with advanced, disseminated disease and are ineligible for surgery.
- A 2-stage system has been used to classify SCLC, based on the ability to include all disease within the field for external-beam radiation therapy:

  – Limited disease
  – Extensive disease

- *Limited Disease (corresponding to stage I-IIIB)*: tumour confined to one hemithorax, regional nodes (ipsilateral and contralateral hilar and mediastinal), and ipsilateral supraclavicular nodes.

  – Median survival 15–20 months, 5-year survival 10–13 % [36, 37].

- *Extensive Disease (corresponding to stage IV)*: tumour has spread beyond the boundaries of limited disease (distant metastasis, malignant pleural or pericardial effusions, contralateral supraclavicular nodes).

  – Median survival 8–13 months, 5-year survival 1–2 % [36, 37]

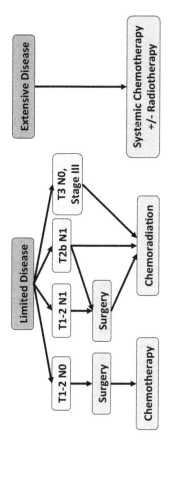

Fɪɢ. 3.5. Management algorithm for small-cell lung cancer.

- Highly sensitive to systemic chemotherapy but with a high rate of relapse [38].

  - Objective response rate: 60–80 %
  - Complete response: 25–50 % of patients with limited disease
  - Platinum-based combinations are often the initial first line chemotherapy regimens with multiple other combinations used as alternative and second-line regimens.

- Thoracic Radiation therapy

  - For management of limited stage disease.
  - Significantly improves local intrathoracic control and provides a small survival advantage when used in addition to chemotherapy [39, 40].

- Surgery

  - Unlike NSCLC, lung resection plays a limited role in the multimodality management of SCLC with no improvement in survival, even for limited stage SCLC [41].
  - However, for very early SCLC, surgery followed by adjuvant platinum-based chemotherapy has been shown to have 5-year survivals as high as 86 % (stage I) and 49 % (stage I and II) and a median overall survival of 47 months (stage I and II) [42, 43].
  - For patients discovered to have node-positive disease on post-operative pathology, adjuvant therapy should also consist of radiation therapy.

- Prophylactic cranial irradiation

  - Brain metastasis is very common in SCLC patients.
  - 18 % of patients have brain metastases at diagnosis, while 80 % will develop brain metastases within 2 years [44, 45].
  - Prophylactic irradiation is associated with a decreased incidence of brain metastases and prolongation of both median disease-free survival and overall survival [46, 47].

# Lung Metastases from Other Primary Tumours

**Overview**

- Lung is a common location for distant metastasis from other primary neoplasms.
- Biologic behaviour of the underlying disease will predict the mechanism of dissemination, pattern of metastasis and aggressiveness.
- Although new pulmonary lesions in a patient with a known primary tumour are highly indicative of metastases (especially where they are multiple), they can also be incidental findings of benign lung lesions or a new metachronous lung cancer (especially when there is a new solitary lung lesion in the absence of any extra-thoracic metastasis) [48].

**Surgical Metastasectomy**

- Given that the prognosis of patients with metastases to the lungs is highly heterogeneous, pulmonary resection may improve long-term survival for a subset of patients.
- For a select group of patients whose primary tumour is under control, pulmonary metastasectomy is feasible and safe.
- Clear communication, possibly including multidisciplinary oncology rounds discussion, with the referring oncologist regarding strategy of resection and systemic therapy, should be undertaken in all patients.
- Several factors can predict a favourable prognosis post-metastasectomy [49, 50]:

  - *Resectability:* a complete resection has been shown to be an independent prognostic factor.

    - Patients should be medically fit with adequate pulmonary reserve to tolerate a resection.

  - *Disease-Free Interval:* a longer disease-free interval (>36 months) is associated with less aggressive behaviour and a greater likelihood of cure following lung resection.

- *Histopathology:* colon cancers, germ cell tumours, sarcomas, breast cancers and well-differentiated thyroid cancers have shown long-term benefit [51–54]. Even certain tumours that are considered to have an aggressive disease course (such as esophageal cancer) have demonstrated a survival advantage in select cases [55, 56].
- *Number of Metastatic Lesions:* patients with more than 1 nodule have decreased survival; however there is no absolute number of metastases that differentiate between surgical and medical disease. With favourable resectability, disease free interval, histopathology and cardiopulmonary fitness, multiple and bilateral metastases may certainly be resected.
- *Low Tumour Burden*

- All aforementioned factors should be taken into consideration by a multidisciplinary tumour board to decide if a patient is a surgical candidate.
- Disseminated disease is typically considered a contraindication, although certain cases of colon cancer with lung and liver metastases are amenable to metastasectomy.
- Non-anatomic wedge resections are typically performed due to the high risk of other pulmonary recurrent metastatic lesions and the need for subsequent resections, as well as the lower risk of lymph node recurrence due to secondary metastatic pulmonary tumours. Albeit rare, the presence of lymph node metastases in the mediastinum due to secondary pulmonary neoplastic disease is generally considered a contraindication to resection due to poor prognosis.

# Section 2: Tracheal Disorders

## Tracheal Cancer

### Epidemiology and Histopathology

- Rare tumours (<0.1 % of all neoplasms) [57].
- >90 % malignant; most commonly squamous-cell carcinoma (45 %) and adenoid cystic carcinoma (25 %) [58].

- High association with smoking (77 %), particularly squamous-cell carcinoma (>90 %) [58]
- Adenoid cystic carcinoma:

  - Resectable: 5-year and 10-year survival 52 % and 29 % [59]
  - Unresectable: 5-year and 10-year survival 33 % and 10 % [59]

- Squamous-cell carcinoma:

  - Resectable: 5-year and 10-year survival 39 % and 18 % [59]
  - Unresectable: 5-year and 10-year survival 7 % and 5 % [59]

**Clinical Presentation and Workup**

- Obstructive symptoms: chronic cough, dyspnea (especially after exertion), stridor, postural-wheezing, post-obstructive pneumonia, respiratory failure.

  - Symptoms develop after lumen obstruction >50–75 %.
  - 8 mm lumen diameter: dyspnea on exertion [60]
  - <5 mm lumen diameter: dyspnea at rest [60]

- Haemoptysis
- Symptoms of local invasion: hoarseness
- Often patients are mis-diagnosed as having adult-onset asthma or COPD, especially with a history of smoking.
- All patients should undergo CT neck/chest/abdomen, bronchoscopy and esophagogastroscopy for detailed characterization and tissue diagnosis.

**Management (Fig. 3.6)**

- Since the best chance for cure is tracheal resection with or without adjuvant radiotherapy, as opposed to definitive chemoradiation [57], patients should undergo evaluation to determine if their tumour is resectable.
- Resectability is determined by tumour location, length and invasion of adjacent structures.

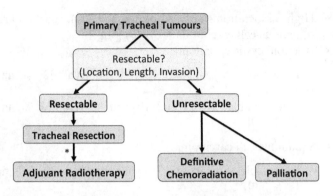

Fig. 3.6. Management algorithm for primary tracheal tumours. *Patients with R1 or R2 resections or squamous-cell histopathology should undergo adjuvant radiotherapy.*

- – The benefits of performing an oncologically sound en-bloc resection with negative margins should be weighed against the risk of dehiscence, which has high rates of mortality.

- Radiotherapy is reserved for unresectable tumours as well as adjuvant therapy for most patients, especially R1/R2 resections and squamous-cell carcinomas.
- Chemotherapy is reserved for unresectable and end-stage disease.
- Palliative options include bronchoscopic debulking (including laser ablation), stents, chemotherapy.

## Tracheal Stenosis

### Overview

- Most commonly a circumferential lesion caused by prolonged intubation with pressure necrosis from the endotracheal tube cuff.
- Other etiologies:

  - – Tracheal cancers
  - – Iatrogenic: mostly after intubation

- External compression: thyroid mass (goitre), vascular rings, aneurysms of the innominate artery, large mediastinal masses, secondary neoplasms
- Inflammatory: Wegner's granulomatosis, systemic polychondritis, amyloidosis
- Infection: tuberculosis, histoplasmosis
- Congenital

- Injury to the cricoid cartilage may involve the larynx, leading to subglottic stenosis. Lesions in the larynx should be managed first before addressing the trachea.

**Presentation**

- Symptoms of airway obstruction: dyspnea, stridor, wheezing, cough, recurrent pneumonias.

  - Patients often mis-diagnosed as having adult-onset asthma or COPD.

**Management**

- *Acute airway obstruction:*

  - Use of inhaled agents for anaesthesia, and avoiding muscle relaxants.
  - Rigid bronchoscopy for complete evaluation of the proximal and distal ends, followed by serial dilations and placement of the endotracheal tube.
  - Other adjuncts: racemic epinephrine, steroids, bronchodilators and heliox.

- Management for patients with significant airway obstructive symptoms is segmental tracheal resection with primary anastomosis.

  - Prior to surgery, patients should be weaned off steroids and given adequate time for mucosal healing of the trachea. Their nutritional status and medical comorbidities should also be optimised, and surgery should be ideally postponed until the patient has recovered from the initial illness that required endotracheal intubation.

- Stents should be avoided if possible to prevent exacerbating the injury and avoiding granulation.

## *Tracheoesophageal Fistula: Acquired*

**Aetiology**

- Benign: iatrogenic (chronic stent erosion, endoscopic procedures, surgeries in the neck), prolonged mechanical ventilation (especially with concomitant nasogastric tube placement), trauma, radiation, infections, granulomatous diseases, diverticula perforation, caustic injury
- Malignant: esophageal (most common), lung, tracheal cancers
- Most fistulas between the oesophagus and airways are tracheoesophageal (55 %) or bronchoesophageal (40 %), while the remainder involve the peripheral lung parenchyma [61].

**Clinical Presentation and Workup**

- Chronic cough, increased secretions
- Aspiration and recurrent pneumonias
- Patients who are mechanically ventilated will manifest a significant air leak through the system (e.g. over-distended stomach, inspiration and expiration tidal volume mismatch).
- Diagnosis is confirmed via barium swallow, bronchoscopy and esophagoscopy.

  - Biopsies should be obtained when malignancy is suspected.
  - Fistula anatomy should be clearly defined to guide management.

**Management**

- Unstable patients should undergo resuscitation (+/– airway control), with fistula control. Once stabilised, early repair should be undertaken.

- Ventilator-dependent patients should ideally be weaned from mechanical ventilation prior to operative intervention to avoid compromising the suture line. However, many do not consider this an absolute contraindication to surgery [62].
- Surgery for benign disease:

  - Options depend on the aetiology and include primary repair of the tracheal and esophageal defects, segmental resection of the trachea with anastomosis and esophagectomy.

    Most common procedure for benign disease is tracheal resection with primary anastomosis and primary closure of the oesophagus as a single-stage procedure.

  - A pedicled interposition tissue flap is typically buttressed to prevent recurrence or dehiscence.

    Options include intercostal muscle, strap muscle, omentum, pericardial fat and pleura.

  - Underlying pathologies should be addressed during surgery.
  - Most patients also require a jejunostomy for enteric feeding.
  - Operative mortality: 5 % [62]

- Surgery for malignant disease: *See* Chap. 3: *Lung and Airway Disorders (Tracheal Cancer)*
- Stents:

  - Either single or double stenting of the trachea and oesophagus
  - Benign disease

    High rates of recurrence and migration; therefore they should not be substituted for definitive surgical treatment.

    Instead, used as a bridge to surgery for patients being weaned off mechanical ventilation.

– Malignant disease:

  Since patients with fistulas have end-stage malignancies, the goal of management is palliation. These
  patients with low-life expectancy benefit significantly
  from stents. The choice of esophageal or airway
  stenting depends on tumour location.

## Tracheal Resection: General Principles

- Anaesthesia should be induced using inhaled agents, while
  avoiding muscle relaxants.
- Blood supply of the trachea enters laterally:

  – Upper trachea: inferior thyroid arteries
  – Branches of the subclavian, innominate, intercostal and
    internal mammary arteries
  – Lower trachea: bronchial arteries

- Unless a tension-free anastomosis can be performed, surgical resection should not be attempted due to high rates
  of mortality. Dehiscence presents weeks after surgery with
  a wound infection and significant subcutaneous emphysema. An R1/R2 resection is preferred over resection with
  too much tension.
- Several mobilisation techniques can be used to allow up to
  50 % of the trachea to be resected safely:

  – Cervical flexion
  – Pre-tracheal dissection
  – Laryngeal release
  – Hilar release

- Mortality: <5 %.

## Tracheostomy

- Tracheostomy provides patients with improved comfort,
  decreased analgesia and weaning from the ventilator.
  Patients also have improved airway security, pulmonary

TABLE 3.2. Indications and contraindications for tracheostomy [64–69].

---

*Indications*
- Supraglottic or glottic pathologic condition
- Neck trauma with severe injury to thyroid or cricoid cartilages, hyoid bone, or great vessels
- Severe facial fractures with risk of upper airway obstruction
- Edema from trauma, burn, infection, or anaphylaxis
- Prophylaxis (e.g. before extensive head and neck procedures)
- Prolonged intubation or expected prolonged intubation (>7 days)
- Recurrent aspiration or inadequate cough reflex requiring regular pulmonary toilet

*Absolute contraindications: none*

*Relative contraindications*
- Prior neck surgery or tracheostomy
- Morbid obesity, short neck
- Thyroid enlargement
- Coagulopathy

---

toilet, oral hygiene and speech, with a decreased risk of subglottic stenosis, vocal cord injury or sinusitis.
- Mortality: <1 % [63]
- Morbidity: 4–10 %
- Indications and contraindications are listed in Table 3.2.

**Open Tracheostomy**

- Position patient supine with neck extended, while under general anaesthesia.
- Make a transverse skin incision 1–2 cm above the suprasternal notch and below the cricoid cartilage.
- Divide the platysma transversely until the midline strap muscles are reached.
- Separate the strap muscles in the midline to identify the pretracheal fascia.
- Divide the thyroid isthmus or reflect it superiorly with retractors to approach the anterior trachea.
- Count the tracheal rings from the cricoid cartilage, and place stay sutures laterally at the second or third tracheal ring.

- The anaesthesiologist should minimise oxygen concentration ($FiO_2$) before incising the ring interspace with a scalpel (number 15 blade). Electrosurgery should not be used to avoid creating a fire.
- Dilate the ring interspace with a tracheal dilator.
- Place a lubricated and pre-tested tracheostomy tube into the airway and rotate it into its proper position under direct visualisation.
- Confirm ventilation with the anaesthesiologist using auscultation, end-tidal $pCO_2$, and possibly bronchoscopy.
- Secure the tracheostomy appliance to the skin with sutures.

**Percutaneous Tracheostomy—Seldinger's Technique**

- Position patient supine with neck extended, under general anaesthesia.
- Under direct vision with bronchoscopy, pull the endotracheal tube back to the larynx, without extubating the patient.
- While visualising the first tracheal ring, insert an 18-gauge needle between the 1st and 2nd tracheal rings.
- Insert a guide wire and remove the needle.
- Make a 1 cm transverse skin incision.
- Dilate the track using sequential dilators and one large dilator.
- Pass the tracheostomy over the guide wire after being loaded over an appropriately sized dilator.
- Verify the tracheostomy position by passing the bronchoscope through the tracheostomy.
- Secure the tracheostomy appliance to the skin with sutures.

**Immediate Complications**

- Haemorrhage
- Apnea
- Pneumothorax/pneumomediastinum
- Pulmonary edema after relieving upper airway obstruction (rarely)

**Early (<48 h) Complications**

- Haemorrhage (after coughing spell while waking from anaesthesia)
- Mucus plug
- Tracheitis
- Subcutaneous emphysema

**Late (>48 h) Complications**

- Infection
- Tracheoinnominate fistula
- Tracheomalacia (especially if an inappropriate-sized cuff is used)
- Laryngeal stenosis (weeks)
- Tracheoesophageal fistula (weeks)

**Post-Decannulation Complications**

- Non-healing fistula
- Infection

**Phonation and Swallowing**

- May resume once the patient is not requiring ventilator support, is awake and has a deflated cuff.
- Passy-Muir valves: one-way valve that opens during inspiration and automatically occludes with exhalation.
- Swallowing difficulty arises due to patients' difficulty in elevating their trachea.
- Extensive swallowing assessment is required to assess aspiration risk.

**Decannulation Criteria (Fig. 3.7)**

- Awake and breathing spontaneously without ventilator support
- Not requiring frequent suctioning
- Satisfactory cough and ability to clear tracheal secretions
- Tracheostomy size 6 or smaller
- No respiratory distress while the tracheostomy is corked

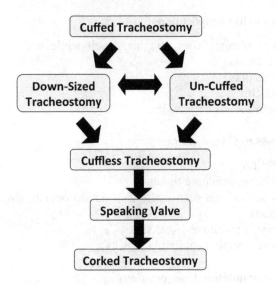

Fig. 3.7. Sequence of steps for tracheostomy decannulation.

**<u>Although decannulation is not required before discharging a patient from a monitored setting (e.g. intensive care unit), patients should not be transferred until they have an un-cuffed tracheostomy, or a cuffless tracheostomy [70].</u>**

- This is to prevent complete airway obstruction and subsequent asphyxiation from mucus plugs.

## Section 3: Miscellaneous Disorders

### *Haemoptysis*

- Classified as massive (>600 mL/24 h) versus non-massive haemoptysis (<600 mL/24 h).
- Life-threatening haemoptysis however can occur with much smaller amounts, particularly in patients with poor cough.

**Pathogenesis**

- Bronchial blood supply (almost always the source) is systemic at high pressure causing significant haemoptysis compared to the low-pressure pulmonary system.
- Bronchial blood supply is nutritive, and is increased in states of persistent inflammation.
- Dead space volume is only 200 mL. Therefore, massive haemoptysis can lead to gas exchange impairment and asphyxia.
- Most common cause is infection causing bronchitis or pneumonia. Other common causes include lung malignancies, tuberculosis, bronchiectasis, and trauma.
- Important to be differentiated from hematemesis or epistaxis on history and physical examination.

**Differential Diagnosis: (* = most common causes)**

- Airways

    - Acute or chronic bronchitis* (chronic bronchitis most common cause)
    - Bronchiectasis*
    - Bronchial carcinoid
    - Malignant airway tumour (*See* Chap. 3: *Tracheal Disorders*)

- Parenchyma

    - Bronchogenic carcinoma*
    - TB
    - Lung abscess
    - Pneumonia—usually gram-negative (e.g. Klebsiella), Staphylococcus, or fungal
    - Idiopathic pulmonary haemosiderosis—idiopathic, parenchymal haemorrhage & infiltrates, Fe-deficiency, haemosiderin-laden macrophages
    - Pulmonary metastasis (renal cell, melanoma)

- Vascular
  - Pulmonary embolism (PE)
  - Increased pulmonary venous pressure (LV failure, mitral stenosis)
  - Arteriovenous malformations
  - Vasculitis—Goodpasture's, Wegener's
  - Pulmonary hypertension
- Miscellaneous
  - Coagulopathy
  - Trauma
  - Foreign body
  - Cystic fibrosis
  - Broncholithiasis
  - Pulmonary endometriosis

**Clinical Approach: (presentation is highly variable depending on aetiology)**

- *History*: Ask about quantity, duration and previous episodes of haemoptysis, history of chronic sputum production (bronchitis, bronchiectasis) or purulent sputum (lung abscess), age (consider carcinoid in young patients), constitutional symptoms, smoking history (lung cancer), pleuritic chest pain (PE, pleural lesion), orthopnea, paroxysmal nocturnal dyspnea (congestive heart failure), rule out epistaxis & hematemesis.
- *Physical Examination*: adenopathy, hoarseness, superior vena cava syndrome, hepatomegaly (cancer), pleural friction rub (PE, pleural lesion), RV heave, split S2 (pulmonary hypertension, mitral stenosis, Eisenmenger's, recurrent PE), localised wheeze (airway tumour), murmur over lung field (AVM).
- *Chest X-Ray* (CXR): ring shadows, air bronchograms (bronchiectasis), air-fluid level (abscess), mass (neoplasm), right ventricle or pulmonary artery prominence (pulmonary hypertension).

**Management of Life-Threatening Haemoptysis (Fig. 3.8)**

- Obtain IV access, perform CXR, history and physical.
- Place patient with suspected bleeding side down (pillow under opposite side).
- Determine ability of patient to expectorate and protect airway; if no (i.e. patient unable to oxygenate and venti-late, losing consciousness):

  - Place left-sided double lumen endotracheal tube (ETT) emergently.
  - Or, if bleeding coming from the right, place single lumen ETT in left mainstem bronchus.
  - Endotracheal intubation without lung isolation should be avoided.

- Initiate antibiotic therapy for suspected infection.
- Consider CT chest if patient able to protect airway and CXR is equivocal regarding lateralization of bleeding.
- Transfer to ICU or OR urgently.
- Bronchoscopy:

  - Indicated to localise site of bleeding, remove blood, irrigate, ensure double-lumen tube is in good position.
  - However, bronchoscopy is ineffective for removing large clots.

- Operative—rigid bronchoscopy under general anaesthesia:

  - Required emergently if patient unable to expectorate and clear airway.
  - Required urgently if patient stabilised with double-lumen tube and large clot unable to be removed.
  - Goal of OR: rigid bronchoscopy to remove blood in airway, irrigate with ice cold saline with dilute epineph-rine to stop bleeding temporarily, place double lumen ET tube in clear airway.
  - Requires close communication with anaesthetist.
  - Avoid paralytics if possible.

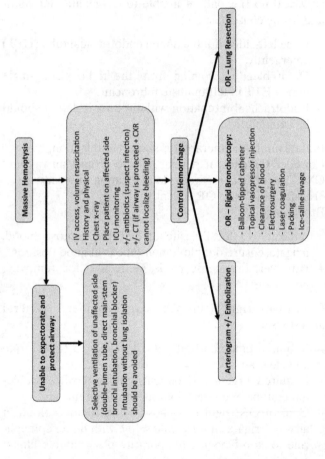

FIG. 3.8. Management algorithm for massive haemoptysis.

- Angiography and bronchial artery embolization:

  - Indicated for life-threatening haemoptysis requiring double-lumen placement where source is infectious or inflammatory.
  - Performed after lung isolation has been accomplished and patient is stabilised.
  - While angiography may reveal an enlarged bronchial vessel, it may appear normal with no active bleeding seen. In such a case, the treating team should still proceed with embolization.

- Operative—pulmonary resection:

  - Rarely indicated for refractory or uncontrolled haemoptysis, where there is clearly a single site of haemorrhage (e.g. apical cavity with bronchial artery aneurysm).

## Lung Abscess

**Pathophysiologic Features that Lead to a Lung Abscess:**

- Aspiration

  - Dental and periodontal disease
  - Alcohol abuse
  - Seizures
  - Neuromuscular disorders with bulbar dysfunction
  - Gastroesophageal Reflux Disease
  - Esophageal dysmotility

- Immunosuppression

  - Congenital
  - Acquired

- Bronchial Obstruction

  - Neoplastic
  - Non-neoplastic

**Microbiology**

- Primary lung abscesses develop from many organisms, mainly anaerobic mouth flora.
- Necrotizing pneumonia forms multiple small cavities in the lung parenchyma.

**Clinical Presentation**

- Patients exhibit symptoms similar to those of pneumonia, which includes coughing, fever, night sweats, haemoptysis, pleuritic chest pain and fatigue.
- Lung abscess should be differentiated from other conditions such as an infected bulla or cavitary tumours.
- Chest x-rays and CT chest show an air-fluid level with a thick wall cavity.
- Location: frequently superior segments of right & left lower lobes, and lateral part of posterior segment of upper lobes (axillary sub-segment). Note that both are adjacent to each other along superior component of major fissure.

**Management**

- Medical management, including chest physiotherapy, expectoration and prolonged antibiotics considered as first-line.
- Failed medical management should undergo drainage:
  - CT-guided drainage shown to be highly effective (85 % success rate with no residual cavity).
- Surgical management is indicated for:
  - Failure of antibiotics and/or CT-guided drainage
  - Abscesses >6 cm, over 6 weeks
  - Bleeding (causing life-threatening haemoptysis)
  - Necrotizing infections with multifocal abscesses
  - Abscess with associated pathology requiring surgery (e.g. lung cancer)
  - Inability to rule out cancer
  - Broncho-pleural fistula and lung abscess

- Principles of surgery

  - Lung isolation is critical. Once the cavity is opened, purulent fluid may flood proximal airway.
  - Bronchial artery embolization should be performed prior to OR if history of marked haemoptysis.

## Chronic Obstructive Pulmonary Disease (COPD): Surgical Management

- Surgical options for patients with COPD include:

  - Bullectomy

    For single, large bulla, occupying half of the pleural cavity.
    Patients with recurrent pneumothoraces.

  - Lung volume-reduction surgery (LVRS)
  - Lung transplantation

- Outcomes following LVRS:

  - Highly controversial with increasing evidence demonstrating effectiveness and improved outcomes for severe emphysema, including lung function, exercise capacity and quality of life.
  - Most existing data on the clinical outcomes of LVRS and patient selection for LVRS come from the National Emphysema Treatment Trial (NETT)—a multicenter prospective randomised-controlled trial of patients undergoing LVRS and maximal medical treatment versus patients only receiving maximal medical treatment. However, these outcomes have also been replicated in studies outside of NETT [71, 72].
  - Lung function: improved BODE index (multidimensional predictor of survival in COPD), FEV1, maximum ventilation rate, tidal volume, total lung capacity, Borg dyspnea score, exercise tolerance (6-min walk test), total sleep time, sleep efficiency and annual rates of COPD exacerbations, with improved outcomes in

patients with upper-lobe-predominant disease and low exercise capacity [73–78].

- Survival: 98 % (95%CI 0.94–1) at 1 year; 95 % (95%CI 0.88–1) at 3 years [73]. Subgroup analysis shows that while patients with a high-risk surgical profile have significantly higher probability of death during the first 3 years of follow-up, mortality rates favoured surgical treatment during subsequent follow-up [79].

- Quality of life scores: significantly higher quality of life scores and quality-adjusted life years (QALY) up to 6 years amongst patients undergoing LVRS and maximal medical treatment ($N = 608$), compared to patients only receiving maximal medical treatment ($N = 610$) [80]. Patients in this trial followed significant preoperative rehabilitation and screening for inclusion: (1) radiographic evidence of bilateral emphysema, (2) severe airflow obstruction and hyperinflation, (3) completion of rehabilitation. Patients at high risk of perioperative morbidity or with contraindications for LVRS were excluded.

- Indications for LVRS:

  - There currently exists no established guideline for LVRS patient referral. The following patients have favourable outcomes and tend to be selected in clinical trials for LVRS [73, 81, 82]:
  - Severe emphysematous destruction and hyperinflation
  - Body-mass index <32
  - FEV1 <45 % (predicted) and >15 % (predicted) if age >70
  - TLC >100 % (predicted)
  - RV >150 % (predicted)
  - $pCO_2$ <60 mmHg at rest on room air
  - $pO_2$ >45 mmHg at rest on room air
  - Marked restriction in quality of life and activities of daily living after failure of maximal medical treatment
  - Heterogeneous distribution with obvious target areas
  - Ability to complete preoperative pulmonary rehabilitation programme
  - Abstinence from smoking >6 months

- Despite these criteria, very few COPD patients are candidates for surgery. Contraindications for LVRS:

  - Major medical co-morbidities, advanced age or poor performance status
  - Pulmonary hypertension (>35 mmHg mean, or >45 mmHg peak pulmonary arterial pressure)
  - Inability to participate in pulmonary rehabilitation
  - Tobacco use
  - Pleural or interstitial disease precluding surgery (e.g. bronchiectasis, lung cancer)
  - Poor exercise capacity following rehabilitation programme (<140 m on 6-min walk test)
  - Diffuse emphysema
  - Previous lung transplant
  - Oxygen requirement >6 L to keep saturation >90 % with exercise

- Support for LVRS programme:

  - Cost: the cost-effectiveness of LVRS compared to medical therapy alone is estimated at USD$140,000 (95 % CI $40,155–$239,359) per QALY gained at 5 years (USD$77,000 for patients with upper-lobe-predominant disease), with a projection of USD$54,000 per QALY at 10 years [83]. While LVRS is more costly per person in the short-term, the long-term value and economic impact may prove otherwise.
  - Medical support for a LVRS programme: because the majority of COPD patients are not candidates for LVRS, enormous medical support is required for a LVRS programme to help handle the volume of referrals to screen the minority of patients eligible for surgery.
  - Given the associated cost and resources required to run a LVRS programme and the perioperative morbidity for LVRS, significant controversy exists regarding the establishment of guidelines for patient referral, as well as the adoption of LVRS across institutions.

# References

1. U.S. Cancer Statistics Working Group – United States Cancer Statistics: 1999–2010 Incidence and Mortality Web-based Report.
2. Canadian Cancer Society – Lung Cancer Statistics.
3. Bach PB et al. Variations in lung cancer risk among smokers. J Natl Cancer Inst. 2003;95(6):470–8.
4. Ettinger DS, Aisner J. Changing face of small-cell lung cancer: real and artifact. J Clin Oncol. 2006;24(28):4526–7.
5. Rigler LG. An overview of cancer of the lung. Semin Roentgenol. 1977;12(3):161–4.
6. Silvestri GA et al. Noninvasive staging of non-small cell lung cancer: ACCP evidenced-based clinical practice guidelines (2nd edition). Chest. 2007;132(3 Suppl):178S–201.
7. Patz Jr EF et al. Thoracic nodal staging with PET imaging with 18FDG in patients with bronchogenic carcinoma. Chest. 1995;108(6):1617–21.
8. Fischer BM, Mortensen J, Hojgaard L. Positron emission tomography in the diagnosis and staging of lung cancer: a systematic, quantitative review. Lancet Oncol. 2001;2(11):659–66.
9. Vansteenkiste JF, Stroobants SS. PET scan in lung cancer: current recommendations and innovation. J Thorac Oncol. 2006; 1(1):71–3.
10. Bou-Assaly W, Pernicano P, Hoeffner E. Systemic air embolism after transthoracic lung biopsy: a case report and review of literature. World J Radiol. 2010;2(5):193–6.
11. Yao X et al. Fine-needle aspiration biopsy versus core-needle biopsy in diagnosing lung cancer: a systematic review. Curr Oncol. 2012;19(1):e16–27.
12. Paone G et al. Endobronchial ultrasound-driven biopsy in the diagnosis of peripheral lung lesions. Chest. 2005;128(5):3551–7.
13. Yasufuku K et al. Endobronchial ultrasound guided transbronchial needle aspiration for staging of lung cancer. Lung Cancer. 2005;50(3):347–54.
14. Gu P et al. Endobronchial ultrasound-guided transbronchial needle aspiration for staging of lung cancer: a systematic review and meta-analysis. Eur J Cancer. 2009;45(8):1389–96.
15. Eloubeidi MA et al. Endoscopic ultrasound-guided fine needle aspiration of mediastinal lymph node in patients with suspected lung cancer after positron emission tomography and computed tomography scans. Ann Thorac Surg. 2005;79(1):263–8.

16. Detterbeck FC et al. Invasive mediastinal staging of lung cancer: ACCP evidence-based clinical practice guidelines (2nd edition). Chest. 2007;132(3 Suppl):202S–20.
17. Tan BB et al. The solitary pulmonary nodule. Chest. 2003;123(1 Suppl):89S–96.
18. Ost D, Fein AM, Feinsilver SH. Clinical practice. The solitary pulmonary nodule. N Engl J Med. 2003;348(25):2535–42.
19. National Cancer Institute: Non-Small Cell Lung Cancer Treatment. [cited 2015 January 26, 2015]; 2014. http://www.cancer.gov/cancertopics/pdq/treatment/non-small-cell-lung/healthprofessional/page4.
20. Pignon JP et al. Lung adjuvant cisplatin evaluation: a pooled analysis by the LACE Collaborative Group. J Clin Oncol. 2008;26(21):3552–9.
21. Winton T et al. Vinorelbine plus cisplatin vs. observation in resected non-small-cell lung cancer. N Engl J Med. 2005;352(25): 2589–97.
22. Arriagada R et al. Cisplatin-based adjuvant chemotherapy in patients with completely resected non-small-cell lung cancer. N Engl J Med. 2004;350(4):351–60.
23. Strauss GM et al. Adjuvant paclitaxel plus carboplatin compared with observation in stage IB non-small-cell lung cancer: CALGB 9633 with the Cancer and Leukemia Group B, Radiation Therapy Oncology Group, and North Central Cancer Treatment Group Study Groups. J Clin Oncol. 2008;26(31):5043–51.
24. Douillard JY et al. Adjuvant vinorelbine plus cisplatin versus observation in patients with completely resected stage IB-IIIA non-small-cell lung cancer (Adjuvant Navelbine International Trialist Association [ANITA]): a randomised controlled trial. Lancet Oncol. 2006;7(9):719–27.
25. PORT Meta-analysis Trialists Group. Postoperative radiotherapy in non-small-cell lung cancer: systematic review and meta-analysis of individual patient data from nine randomised controlled trials. Lancet. 1998;352(9124):257–63.
26. Thomas M et al. Effect of preoperative chemoradiation in addition to preoperative chemotherapy: a randomised trial in stage III non-small-cell lung cancer. Lancet Oncol. 2008;9(7):636–48.
27. Higgins K et al. Preoperative chemotherapy versus preoperative chemoradiotherapy for stage III (N2) non-small-cell lung cancer. Int J Radiat Oncol Biol Phys. 2009;75(5):1462–7.
28. van Meerbeeck JP et al. Randomized controlled trial of resection versus radiotherapy after induction chemotherapy in stage

IIIA-N2 non-small-cell lung cancer. J Natl Cancer Inst. 2007; 99(6):442–50.

29. Albain KS et al. Radiotherapy plus chemotherapy with or without surgical resection for stage III non-small-cell lung cancer: a phase III randomised controlled trial. Lancet. 2009;374(9687): 379–86.

30. de Cabanyes Candela S, Detterbeck FC. A systematic review of restaging after induction therapy for stage IIIa lung cancer: prediction of pathologic stage. J Thorac Oncol. 2010;5(3):389–98.

31. Marra A et al. Remediastinoscopy in restaging of lung cancer after induction therapy. J Thorac Cardiovasc Surg. 2008;135(4): 843–9.

32. Ginsberg RJ, Rubinstein LV. Randomized trial of lobectomy versus limited resection for T1 N0 non-small cell lung cancer. Lung Cancer Study Group. Ann Thorac Surg. 1995;60(3):615–22. discussion 622–3.

33. Landreneau RJ et al. Wedge resection versus lobectomy for stage I (T1 N0 M0) non-small-cell lung cancer. J Thorac Cardiovasc Surg. 1997;113(4):691–8. discussion 698–700.

34. Chen FF et al. Video-assisted thoracoscopic surgery lobectomy versus open lobectomy in patients with clinical stage non-small cell lung cancer: a meta-analysis. Eur J Surg Oncol. 2013;39(9): 957–63.

35. Rusch VW et al. The IASLC lung cancer staging project: a proposal for a new international lymph node map in the forthcoming seventh edition of the TNM classification for lung cancer. J Thorac Oncol. 2009;4(5):568–77.

36. Osterlind K et al. Long-term disease-free survival in small-cell carcinoma of the lung: a study of clinical determinants. J Clin Oncol. 1986;4(9):1307–13.

37. Seifter EJ, Ihde DC. Therapy of small cell lung cancer: a perspective on two decades of clinical research. Semin Oncol. 1988; 15(3):278–99.

38. Hann CL, Rudin CM. Management of small-cell lung cancer: incremental changes but hope for the future. Oncology (Williston Park). 2008;22(13):1486–92.

39. Pignon JP et al. A meta-analysis of thoracic radiotherapy for small-cell lung cancer. N Engl J Med. 1992;327(23):1618–24.

40. Warde P, Payne D. Does thoracic irradiation improve survival and local control in limited-stage small-cell carcinoma of the lung? A meta-analysis. J Clin Oncol. 1992;10(6):890–5.

41. Lad T et al. A prospective randomized trial to determine the benefit of surgical resection of residual disease following response of small cell lung cancer to combination chemotherapy. Chest. 1994;106(6 Suppl):320S–3.
42. Brock MV et al. Surgical resection of limited disease small cell lung cancer in the new era of platinum chemotherapy: Its time has come. J Thorac Cardiovasc Surg. 2005;129(1):64–72.
43. Bischof M et al. Surgery and chemotherapy for small cell lung cancer in stages I-II with or without radiotherapy. Strahlenther Onkol. 2007;183(12):679–84.
44. Nugent JL et al. CNS metastases in small cell bronchogenic carcinoma: increasing frequency and changing pattern with lengthening survival. Cancer. 1979;44(5):1885–93.
45. Seute T et al. Neurologic disorders in 432 consecutive patients with small cell lung carcinoma. Cancer. 2004;100(4):801–6.
46. Meert AP et al. Prophylactic cranial irradiation in small cell lung cancer: a systematic review of the literature with meta-analysis. BMC Cancer. 2001;1:5.
47. Slotman B et al. Prophylactic cranial irradiation in extensive small-cell lung cancer. N Engl J Med. 2007;357(7):664–72.
48. Madani et al. Clinical significance of incidental pulmonary nodules in esophageal cancer patients. J Gastrointest Surg. 2014;18(2):226–32.
49. Casiraghi M et al. A 10-year single-center experience on 708 lung metastasectomies: the evidence of the "international registry of lung metastases". J Thorac Oncol. 2011;6(8):1373–8.
50. The International Registry of Lung Metastases. Long-term results of lung metastasectomy: prognostic analyses based on 5206 cases. J Thorac Cardiovasc Surg. 1997;113(1):37–49.
51. Friedel G et al. Results of lung metastasectomy from breast cancer: prognostic criteria on the basis of 467 cases of the International Registry of Lung Metastases. Eur J Cardiothorac Surg. 2002;22(3):335–44.
52. Younes RN, Abrao F, Gross J. Pulmonary metastasectomy for colorectal cancer: long-term survival and prognostic factors. Int J Surg. 2013;11(3):244–8.
53. Porterfield JR et al. Thoracic metastasectomy for thyroid malignancies. Eur J Cardiothorac Surg. 2009;36(1):155–8.
54. Protopapas AD et al. Thoracic metastasectomy in thyroid malignancies. Ann Thorac Surg. 2001;72(6):1906–8.
55. Kozu Y et al. Surgical treatment for pulmonary metastases from esophageal carcinoma after definitive chemoradiotherapy: experience from a single institution. J Cardiothorac Surg. 2011;6:135.

56. Shiono S et al. Disease-free interval length correlates to prognosis of patients who underwent metastasectomy for esophageal lung metastases. J Thorac Oncol. 2008;3(9):1046–9.
57. Macchiarini P. Primary tracheal tumours. Lancet Oncol. 2006; 7(1):83–91.
58. Webb BD et al. Primary tracheal malignant neoplasms: the University of Texas MD Anderson Cancer Center experience. J Am Coll Surg. 2006;202(2):237–46.
59. Gaissert HA et al. Long-term survival after resection of primary adenoid cystic and squamous cell carcinoma of the trachea and carina. Ann Thorac Surg. 2004;78(6):1889–96. discussion 1896–7.
60. Hollingsworth HM. Wheezing and stridor. Clin Chest Med. 1987;8(2):231–40.
61. Hurtgen M, Herber SC. Treatment of malignant tracheoesophageal fistula. Thorac Surg Clin. 2014;24(1):117–27.
62. Shen KR et al. Surgical management of acquired nonmalignant tracheoesophageal and bronchoesophageal fistulae. Ann Thorac Surg. 2010;90(3):914–8. discussion 919.
63. Walts PA, Murthy SC, DeCamp MM. Techniques of surgical tracheostomy. Clin Chest Med. 2003;24(3):413–22.
64. Heffner JE. Tracheotomy application and timing. Clin Chest Med. 2003;24(3):389–98.
65. Heffner JE, Hess D. Tracheostomy management in the chronically ventilated patient. Clin Chest Med. 2001;22(1):55–69.
66. Ernst A, Critchlow J. Percutaneous tracheostomy-special considerations. Clin Chest Med. 2003;24(3):409–12.
67. de Boisblanc BP. Percutaneous dilational tracheostomy techniques. Clin Chest Med. 2003;24(3):399–407.
68. MacIntyre NR et al. Evidence-based guidelines for weaning and discontinuing ventilatory support: a collective task force facilitated by the American College of Chest Physicians; the American Association for Respiratory Care; and the American College of Critical Care Medicine. Chest. 2001;120(6 Suppl):375S–95.
69. Henderson JJ et al. Difficult Airway Society guidelines for management of the unanticipated difficult intubation. Anaesthesia. 2004;59(7):675–94.
70. Fernandez R et al. Intensive care unit discharge to the ward with a tracheostomy cannula as a risk factor for mortality: a prospective, multicenter propensity analysis. Crit Care Med. 2011;39(10): 2240–5.
71. Hillerdal G et al. Comparison of lung volume reduction surgery and physical training on health status and physiologic outcomes:

a randomized controlled clinical trial. Chest. 2005;128(5): 3489–99.

72. Zahid I et al. Is lung volume reduction surgery effective in the treatment of advanced emphysema? Interact Cardiovasc Thorac Surg. 2011;12(3):480–6.

73. Ginsburg ME et al. Lung volume reduction surgery using the NETT selection criteria. Ann Thorac Surg. 2011;91(5):1556–60. discussion 1561.

74. Criner GJ et al. Effects of lung volume reduction surgery on gas exchange and breathing pattern during maximum exercise. Chest. 2009;135(5):1268–79.

75. Kozora E et al. Improved neurobehavioral functioning in emphysema patients following lung volume reduction surgery compared with medical therapy. Chest. 2005;128(4):2653–63.

76. Krachman SL et al. Effects of lung volume reduction surgery on sleep quality and nocturnal gas exchange in patients with severe emphysema. Chest. 2005;128(5):3221–8.

77. Washko GR et al. The effect of lung volume reduction surgery on chronic obstructive pulmonary disease exacerbations. Am J Respir Crit Care Med. 2008;177(2):164–9.

78. Naunheim KS et al. Long-term follow-up of patients receiving lung-volume-reduction surgery versus medical therapy for severe emphysema by the National Emphysema Treatment Trial Research Group. Ann Thorac Surg. 2006;82(2):431–43.

79. Kaplan RM et al. Long-term follow-up of high-risk patients in the national emphysema treatment trial. Ann Thorac Surg. 2014; 98(5):1782–9.

80. Kaplan RM, Sun Q, Ries AL. Quality of well-being outcomes in the National Emphysema Treatment Trial. Chest. 2015; 147(2): 377–87.

81. Meyers BF, Patterson GA. Chronic obstructive pulmonary disease. 10: Bullectomy, lung volume reduction surgery, and transplantation for patients with chronic obstructive pulmonary disease. Thorax. 2003;58(7):634–8.

82. Criner GJ et al. The National Emphysema Treatment Trial (NETT) Part II: lessons learned about lung volume reduction surgery. Am J Respir Crit Care Med. 2011;184(8):881–93.

83. Ramsey SD et al. Updated evaluation of the cost-effectiveness of lung volume reduction surgery. Chest. 2007;131(3):823–32.

# Chapter 4
## Pleural Disorders

**Stephen D. Gowing and Amin Madani**

## Anatomy and Physiology

- The pleural cavity is lined by parietal and visceral pleura, which are smooth membranes that are continuous with one another at the hilum and pulmonary ligaments.
- *Parietal Pleura:* innermost chest wall layer, divided into cervical, costal, mediastinal and diaphragmatic pleura.

   – Arterial supply and venous drainage: systemic
   – Highly innervated by intercostal nerves responsible for somatic pain sensation when the parietal pleura is subjected to trauma (e.g. tube thoracostomy, thoracotomy) or tumour invasion
   – Phrenic nerve also innervates the mediastinal and diaphragmatic pleura

S.D. Gowing, M.D.
Department of Surgery, McGill University Health Center,
Montreal, QC, Canada

A. Madani, M.D. (✉)
Department of Surgery, McGill University,
Montreal, QC, Canada
e-mail: amin.madani@mail.mcgill.ca

A. Madani et al. (eds.), *Pocket Manual of General Thoracic Surgery*, DOI 10.1007/978-3-319-17497-6_4,
© Springer International Publishing Switzerland 2015

- *Visceral Pleura:* layer covering both lungs

  - Arterial supply: systemic and pulmonary; venous drainage: pulmonary
  - Innervated by the autonomic nervous system

- The two layers are separated by a thin layer of pleural fluid, which serves to allow transmission of forces from the chest wall to the lungs during inspiration and expiration.

  - Pleural fluid under normal conditions is about 0.25 mL/kg and is plasma-like consistency [1].
  - Pleural fluid turnover: 0.15 mL/kg/h [2].
  - The production and reabsorption of fluid is dictated by the Staling forces of parietal and visceral pleura capillaries (hydrostatic pressure, plasma oncotic pressure), as well as capillary permeability and the negative intrathoracic pressure. The lymphatics also have a significant ability to reabsorb large protein molecules and fluid. Any disruption or alterations of these mechanisms may lead to a pleural effusion.
  - Fluid moves via a net filtration gradient from the parietal pleura capillaries into the pleura, while fluid is reabsorbed generally by parietal pleural lymphatics.
  - The function of the pleural fluid is to decrease friction between the parietal and visceral pleura during respiration, allow apposition of the lungs to the chest wall and ensure coupling between the lung, chest wall and diaphragm to optimise ventilation.

## Pneumothorax

**Overview**

- Abnormal presence of air within the pleural cavity
- Results in dissociation of the parietal and visceral pleura leading to a disruption of lung mechanics.
- Lung compression reduces lung compliance, volumes and diffusion capacity.

TABLE 4.1. Aetiology of pneumothorax.

| | |
|---|---|
| *Spontaneous* | *Primary* |
| | *Secondary* |
| | – Chronic obstructive pulmonary disease |
| | – Bronchiolitis |
| | – Pneumocystis infection |
| | – Cystic fibrosis |
| | – Asthma |
| | – Necrotizing pneumonia |
| | – Tuberculosis infection |
| | – Congenital cysts |
| | – Pulmonary fibrosis |
| | *Catamenial* |
| *Traumatic* | Blunt injury |
| | Penetrating injury |
| *Iatrogenic* | Barotrauma—mechanical ventilation |
| | Thoracentesis |
| | Percutaneous transthoracic lung biopsy |
| | Central venous catheterization |
| | Thoracotomy/thoracostomy |
| *Others* | Bronchopleural fistula |
| | Esophageal perforation |

**Tension Pneumothorax**

- If left untreated, air can accumulate without decompressing adequately, leading to high positive pleural pressures, causing severe lung collapse, and compression of the mediastinum, great vessels and heart, and ultimately haemodynamic compromise.
- Patients in tension pneumothorax require immediate clinical diagnosis, followed by needle decompression in the second intercostal space at the midclavicular line, followed by tube thoracostomy.

**Aetiology (Table 4.1)**

- *Spontaneous Pneumothorax:* no underlying trauma or iatrogenic cause for pneumothorax

- *Primary Spontaneous Pneumothorax:* no known underlying lung disease (Fig. 4.1)
  - Incidence 7.4/100,000 (men) and 1.2/100,000 (women) annually in the USA [3].
  - Caused by rupture of small bleb (bullae) usually in apices of upper or lower lobes, allowing air to leak into the pleural cavity.
  - 80 % of patients will demonstrate emphysema-like changes on CT scan [4].
  - Occur most commonly in thin tall young male patients. Smoking and atmospheric pressures changes are also risk factors [5].

- *Secondary Spontaneous Pneumothorax:* known underlying lung disease.
  - Incidence 6.3/100,000 (men) and 2.0/100,000 (women) annually in the USA [3].
  - Underlying disease causing rupture and air leak

**Clinical Presentation**

- Pleuritic chest pain and dyspnea (most common)
- Physical examination may be normal if the pneumothorax is <25 %.
  - Decreased breath sounds, hyperresonance on the affected side (not always present)
  - Subcutaneous emphysema
  - Tension pneumothorax also presents with tracheal deviation to the contralateral side, severe respiratory distress and haemodynamic instability.
  - Rarely: pneumomediastinum or pneumopericardium (Hamman's sign)

- Diagnosis is established by an upright chest X-ray (Fig. 4.2). If clinical signs of tension physiology are evident, X-ray confirmation should be omitted and immediate decompression should ensue.
  - Expiratory view accentuates the separation of the parietal and visceral pleura.

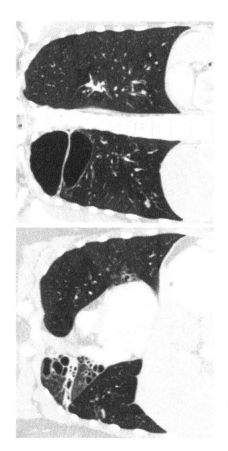

FIG. 4.1. Chest CT of a 27-year-old patient with severe bullous disease. This patient suffered from recurrent primary spontaneous pneumothoraces.

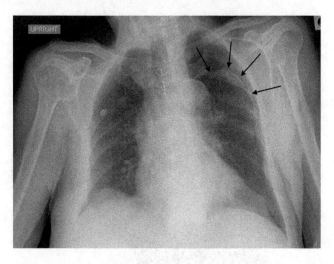

Fig. 4.2. Patient presenting with a traumatic pneumothorax after blunt trauma to the chest. Black arrows denote the outline of the collapsed lung.

- Pneumothorax in supine patients accumulates into the dependent regions of the anterior and subdiaphragmatic pleura and may be detected as a deep sulcus sign.
- Although CT scan is the gold-standard for diagnosis, it is not necessary for the majority of patients with first-episode spontaneous pneumothorax since it does not change the management.
- Ultrasound is also an accurate, rapid and non-invasive test, yet requires operator experience.

  Sensitivity: 95–98 %; true-negative rate: 100 % [6, 7]
  Subcutaneous emphysema can create significant interference.

**Management**

- The aetiology largely dictates both immediate and definitive management.

- *Observation:*
  - Reserved for asymptomatic patients with a small pneumothorax who are unlikely to have an ongoing air leak. Follow-up radiography should be obtained within 24–48 h to document improvement.
  - Supplemental oxygen can help decrease the alveolar pressure of nitrogen in the body, thus creating a gradient to reabsorb the air from the pleura (mostly composed of nitrogen) into the alveoli and tissues.
  - Conservative management re-expands the lung at an average rate of 2.2 %/day with a 79 % success rate [8].
  - Failure for the pneumothorax to resolve may lead to fibrothorax (fibrous entrapment of the lung).

- *Aspiration:*
  - A small cannula can be used to aspirate pleural air, with a success rate of 75 and 40 % for a primary and secondary spontaneous pneumothorax, respectively. This technique is rarely used.
  - Can be attached to a Heimlich one-way valve or a three-way stop-cock with a large syringe [9].

- *Percutaneous Catheters:*
  - Small-calibre tube thoracostomy can be performed percutaneously via the Seldinger technique and attached to either a Heimlich one-way valve or suction.
  - Use is limited to a spontaneous pneumothorax with limited respiratory symptoms.

- *Tube Thoracostomy:*
  - Large-bore chest tubes are the standard-of-care for treatment of traumatic pneumothoraces, unstable patients, persistent or large air leaks and associated effusions or haemothoraces.
  - Clamping of the tube is controversial. If performed, a follow-up chest radiograph should be done in several hours to assess for re-accumulation.

- Outpatient management is acceptable with the use of a Heimlich one-way valve [10].
- Complications of chest tube insertion include: injury to the lung, intercostal vessels, or great vessels, misplacement in the fissures or outside the pleural cavity, infection, and re-expansion pulmonary edema caused with rapid re-expansion leading to increase in capillary permeability.

- The appropriate initial management option should be tailored to the expected size of the air leak.
- Conservative options include observation, needle aspiration, and small-bore tube thoracostomy connected to an underwater seal. For persistent or larger air leaks, large-bore chest tubes with underwater seal connected to wall suction can be used, with surgery and/or pleurodesis as last resorts [11].
- Recurrence after spontaneous pneuothorax is 30 % after the first episode, with the majority occurring within 2 years [12]. Independent risk factors for recurrence include: pulmonary fibrosis, age >60 years, increased height/weight ratio [13]. Recurrence rate increases after each episode.
- *Surgery:*

  - Guidelines recommend waiting at least 3–5 days for resolution of a spontaneous pneumothorax before considering definitive surgical management [14].
  - A bullectomy can be performed preferably via a VATS approach with a success rate >95 % [15]. Other options including open thoracotomy and axillary approaches.
  - Indications for bullectomy [14]:

    After the second spontaneous primary pneumothorax
    After the first spontaneous primary pneumothorax in patients with high-risk professions, or patients exposed to significant changes in atmospheric pressures
    After the first spontaneous secondary pneumothorax

TABLE 4.2. Benign pleural effusions with incidence in the USA [18].

| Causes | Incidence (cases/year) |
|---|---|
| Congestive heart failure | 500,000 |
| Parapneumonic effusion/empyema | 300,000 |
| Pulmonary embolus | 150,000 |
| Viral pleuritis | 100,000 |
| Post-coronary artery bypass graft | 60,000 |
| Hepatic hydrothorax | 50,000 |
| Collagen vascular disease | 6,000 |
| Tuberculosis pleuritis | 2,500 |

- *Pleurodesis:*
  - Although surgery as definitive management of recurrent pneumothoraces is preferred, pleurodesis with talc, bleomycin or doxycycline remains an option with success rates of 75–90 % [16, 17]. *See* Chap. 4*: Pleural Disorders (Pleurodesis Technique).*

## Pleural Effusions

- An abnormal collection of fluid in the pleural space
  - Can be transudative (low protein) or exudative (high protein).
- Benign pleural effusions are twice as common as malignant pleural effusions [18] (Table 4.2).

**Pathophysiology [19]:** *See* **Chap. 4:** *Pleural Disorders (Anatomy and Physiology)*

- Increased pulmonary capillary pressure (CHF, renal failure)
- Increased pulmonary capillary permeability (pneumonia)
- Decreased intrapleural pressure (atelectasis)
- Decreased plasma oncotic pressure (hypoalbuminemia)
- Increased pleural permeability (infection, inflammation)
- Obstruction of pleural lymphatic drainage (malignancy)

- Fluid from other sites or cavities (peritoneum, retroperitoneum)
- Rupture of thoracic vessels (haemothorax, chylothorax)
- Drugs [18]

**Work-Up (Table 4.3)**

- *Serum Laboratory:* blood count and differential (high white count suggests infection, bleeding, malignancy), serum electrolytes, urea, creatinine, liver function tests and liver enzymes, albumin, lactate dehydrogenase, lipase, cardiac enzymes, electrocardiogram
- *Imaging:*

  - Chest X-ray (presence of >250 mL pleural fluid [20])

    Complicated pleural infections are suggested by abnormal pleural indentation that does not correspond to the effects of gravity on pleural fluid.

  - Ultrasound: can identify small effusions and loculations, and can guide thoracocentesis, drain placement and pleural biopsy.
  - CT scan: best imaging study to characterise size, location, presence of loculations and underlying cause of pleural effusions (Fig. 4.3). It can also guide chest drain placement for complicated effusions/empyema.

    Signs of pleural infection include pleural thickening, pleural space air (gas-forming organisms), and the split pleura sign in empyema (pleural fluid encased by distinct thickened visceral and parietal pleura) [21].

- *Pleural Fluid Sampling:* unless the cause of the effusion is known (i.e. CHF) the pleural fluid should be sampled.

  - *Pleural Fluid Characteristics* [22]:

    Straw colour (normal, transudate)
    Turbid/purulent (empyema)
    Blood (trauma, malignancy, parapneumonic)
    Enteric content (esophageal rupture)
    Bile (bilothorax)

TABLE 4.3. Differential diagnosis of pleural effusions.

| *Transudative effusions* | |
| --- | --- |
| Cardiovascular | Congestive heart failure |
| | Pulmonary embolus |
| Infradiaphragmatic | Cirrhosis |
| | Peritoneal dialysis |
| Other | Nephrotic syndrome |
| | Hypoalbuminemia (malnutrition, liver failure) |

| *Exudative effusions* | |
| --- | --- |
| Infections (most common) | Bacterial (sepsis, pneumonia) |
| | Tuberculosis |
| | Viral (respiratory, hepatic, cardiac) |
| | Fungal |
| | Parasitic |
| Neoplasm | Primary lung cancer |
| | Metastatic disease (lung, breast, colon and ovarian cancers most common) |
| | Mesothelioma |
| Infradiaphragmatic | Pancreatitis |
| | Peritonitis |
| | Bilothorax (biliopleural fistula, bile duct obstruction) |
| | Inflammatory bowel disease |
| | Intra-abdominal abscess |
| | Endoscopic esophageal sclerotherapy |
| | Meigs syndrome (pleural effusion and ascites with pelvic tumours) |
| Autoimmune | |
| Drugs | |
| Post-operative | |
| Other | Amyloidosis |
| | Haemothorax |
| | Chylothorax |
| | Esophageal rupture |
| | Benign asbestos-related effusion |

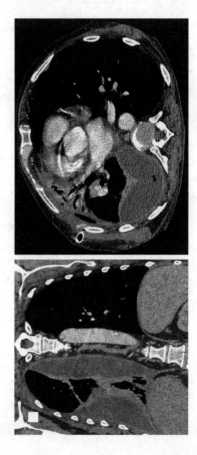

Fig. 4.3. Patient presenting with a parapneumonic effusion that progressed to advanced stage of empyema.

– *Pleural Fluid Analysis:* the following tests should be utilised to characterise the effusion [18, 19]:

pH (<7.2 useful for identifying complicated infected effusions)
LDH (should be measured in pleural fluid and serum)
Protein (pleural fluid and serum)
Bacterial culture (some fluid should be additionally placed in blood culture bottles to improve diagnostic accuracy [23, 24]) and Gram Stain

- Adding pleural fluid to 2 blood culture bottles can increase rates of pathogen identification by approximately 20–60 % [23, 24].

Cytology (to detect malignancy)
CBC (to identify WBCs from infection, or RBCs from blood)
Acid-fast bacilli (AFB) PCR (if lymphocytic effusion is found or TB is a concern especially in endemic regions)

– *Light's Criteria:* used to distinguish exudative from transudative pleural effusions. If 1 or more are positive, effusion is exudative [25].

Pleural Fluid/Serum Protein ratio >0.5
Pleural Fluid/Serum LHD ratio >0.6
Pleural Fluid LDH >2/3 the upper limit of normal serum LDH

- *Pleural Biopsy*: can assist the diagnosis of tuberculosis, malignancy, and amyloidosis when diagnosis is uncertain [26].

# Pleural Infections (Empyema)

- Infection of the pleural space (exudative effusion) [27].
- 70–80 % patients may be managed with non-surgical management (drainage + antibiotics + fibrinolytic therapy) [28, 29].
- Increased incidence in alcoholic and intravenous drug users (risk of aspiration) [30].

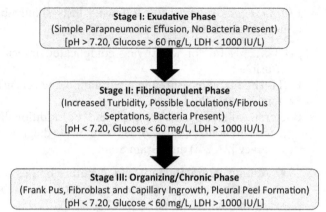

Fig. 4.4. Classification and natural history of empyema.

**Symptoms**

- Similar to pneumonia: pleuritic chest pain, fever, cough, dyspnea, malaise [20]
- Constitutional symptoms (malaise, fatigue, weight loss, anorexia) in malignant pleural effusions

**Causes**

- Direct contamination of pleural space (trauma, surgery)
- Hematologic spread (bacteremia/sepsis)
- Direct extension from lung parenchyma (parapneumonic)
- Rupture of intrapulmonary abscess or infected cavity
- Bronchopleural fistula
- Extension from mediastinum (esophageal perforation)

**Classification**

- Progression through stages occurs over 3–6 weeks (Fig. 4.4) [27, 31].
- Untreated empyema eventually progresses to fibro-thorax [32].

**Microbiology [33]:**

- Community Acquired (85 %):

  – Aerobes (73 %): Streptococci (72 %; S. milleri/anginosus (46 %), S. pneumonia (40 %)), Staphylococci (14 %; MSSA (77 %), MRSA (20 %)), gram-negative (12 %), others (2 %)
  – Anaerobes (22 %)
  – Other (5 %)

- Nosocomial (15 %):

  – Aerobes (88 %): Staphylococci (40 %; MRSA (71 %), MSSA (29 %)), gram-negative (26 %), Streptococci (21 %), Enterococci (13 %)
  – Anaerobes (8 %)
  – Other (4 %)

**Management**

- Drainage:

  – Historically large bore chest tubes (30–36 Fr) were advocated for drainage of pleural infections due to fear of tube blockage by thick viscous drainage [20].
  – A recent case series using 10–16 Fr tubes of pleural infections reported a 72 % success rate, comparable to large bore (>30 Fr) chest tubes [34].
  – A retrospective analysis of 405 patients treated with chest tube drainage of various sizes (<10 Fr, 10–14 Fr, 15–20 Fr, >20 Fr) revealed no difference in mortality or requirement for decortication [35].

    No differences in chest radiograph change following drainage, length of stay or pulmonary function after 3 months were noted between tube size groups.
    Irrigation of pleural cavity can be done with sterile saline following drain insertion, however evidence supporting this practice is lacking [20].

- Antibiotics:
  - Patients often present with signs of sepsis.
  - Broad-spectrum antibiotic therapy covering gram-positive, gram-negative (including Pseudomonas) and anaerobic bacteria is indicated.
  - Focus antibiotics once cultures obtained.
  - Antibiotics in pleural fluid typically reach approximately 75 % of serum levels [20].
  - Duration of antibiotics: minimal evidence suggesting optimal duration, however therapy is generally continued for 2–4 weeks following resolution of signs and symptoms in order to achieve clinical resolution, depending on microbiology, response to therapy, extent of disease, adequacy of drainage and patient factors (e.g. immune status).

- Fibrinolytic Therapy (Streptokinase/tPA +/− DNAse):
  - Used as treatment of loculated parapneumonic effusions and empyema.
  - Aimed to reduce incidence of surgical intervention.
  - Meta-analysis of 7 RCTs comparing fibrinolytic therapy to placebo shows reduction in surgical intervention but not in mortality or length of stay [28].
  - Double-blind RCT MIST2 trial evaluating t-PA and DNAse for patients with pleural infection [36].

    Randomised to 1 of 4 treatments for 3 days: t-PA and DNAse, t-PA and placebo, placebo and DNAse, double placebo.

    Primary outcome: change in pleural opacity (percentage of hemithorax occupied by effusion on chest X-ray [Mean (+/− SD) change in pleural opacity]).

    t-PA + DNAse versus placebo:

    - Change in pleural opacity: $-29.5 \pm 23.3$ % vs. $-17.2 \pm 19.6$ %, $p=0.005$

- Surgical referral at 3 months: OR 0.17; 95 % CI, 0.03 to 0.87; $P=0.03$.
- Hospital stay (mean difference): −6.7 days; 95 % CI, −12.0 to −1.9; $P=0.006$.

Non-significant for t-PA or DNAse alone versus placebo.

- Decortication:

  – Performed by open posterolateral thoracotomy or by VATS
  – Indications:

    Stages II and III after failure of chest tube drainage, intrapleural fibrinolysis and antibiotic therapy.
    Late chronic empyema with entrapped lung.

  – Provides surgical drainage and allows lung to re-expand eliminating potential space that harbours bacteria.
  – Complete decortication allows for lung re-expansion to tamponade air leak and bleeding [20, 27, 32].
  – VATS Decortication (VATSD) versus Open Thoracotomy Decortication (OD):

    Equivalent rates of resolution [37]
    VATSD success rate: 85 % [38]
    VATSD conversion rate to open: 0–3.5 % (early empyema) and 7.1–46 % (late empyema) [38]
    Significantly reduced length of stay, post-operative pain and post-operative complications for VATSD compared to open

**Risk Stratification**

- UK Multicentre Intrapleural Sepsis Trial (MIST) 1 and 2 RAPID Score [39]:

  – 5 factors: age, serum urea, serum albumin, fluid purulence, likely origin of infection
  – Total score out of 7: low, medium and high-risk groups

TABLE 4.4. Differential diagnosis of chylothorax [18, 27, 42].

| | |
|---|---|
| *Traumatic (50 %)* | |
| Iatrogenic | Post-surgical: lymph node dissection, intrathoracic surgery, neck surgery |
| Trauma | Blunt trauma |
| | Penetrating trauma |
| *Medical (44 %)* | |
| Neoplasm (most common non-traumatic cause) | Lymphoma |
| | Lymphoproliferative disorders (CLL) |
| | Esophageal cancer |
| | Mediastinal malignancy |
| | Bronchogenic carcinoma |
| | Metastatic cancer |
| Benign tumours | Retrosternal goitre |
| Infectious diseases altering lymphatic drainage | Tuberculosis |
| | Filariasis |
| | Mediastinitis |
| | Ascending lymphangitis |
| Congenital | Primary lymphatic dysplasia |
| | Lymphangioleiomyomatosis |
| | Intestinal lymphatic dysplasia |
| | Congenital pulmonary lymphangiectasis |
| Other | Amyloidosis |
| | Sarcoidosis |
| | Post-irradiation |
| | Cirrhosis |
| | SVC or central venous thrombosis |
| *Idiopathic (6 %)* | |

   Low-risk (0–2): 5 % mortality risk
   High-risk (5–7): 50 % mortality risk

– Decision-making tool for earlier fibrinolytic therapy versus surgery.

## Chylothorax (Table 4.4)

• A turbid milky white effusion resulting from transection (traumatic) or obstruction of the thoracic duct (TD) or its branches.

- 1.5–2.5 L of lymphatic fluid pass through the TD per day.
- TD leak results in rapid volume, lymphocyte, nutrition, fat-soluble vitamin and electrolyte losses [40].
- TD leak can induce immunosuppression in patients [41].
- 1/200 incidence post-thoracic surgery [18].
- Chylous ascites can also be a source of chylothorax [42].

**Pleural Fluid Investigations**

- Lipoprotein electrophoresis: the presence of chylomicrons confirms chyle leak [43].
- Elevated pleural fluid triglyceride levels (>110 mg/dL).
- CBC and differential demonstrates >80 % lymphocytes [44].

**Thoracic Duct Anatomy**

- Intestinal/Lumbar lymphatics → cysterna chylii (anterior to L1/L2) → aortic hiatus of diaphragm (T12) → right chest (between aorta and azygous vein) → crosses midline at T4 (behind oesophagus) → left posterior mediastinum (behind aorta, left side of oesophagus, behind left subclavian artery) → crosses over left subclavian artery (anterolateral mediastinum) → enters confluence of left jugular and subclavian veins [40].

**Treatment—Traumatic Chylothorax (Post-surgical, Trauma)**

- Pleural Effusion Drainage [27]:
  - Chest tube is used to drain the pleural cavity providing symptomatic relief.
  - Monitoring of drain output (milky colour indicating ongoing chyle leak)
- Dietary Control [27, 40]:
  - Total Parenteral Nutrition (TPN), fasting, or reduced fat diet with Medium Chain Triglyceride (MCT) supplementation.

    MCT are absorbed by intestinal epithelium into the portal venous circulation bypassing lymphatic absorption and decreasing lymphatic flow to allow duct closure.

– Dietary control measures are usually maintained for 1–2 weeks followed by fat challenge (cream or olive oil PO/PT).

Increased milky chest tube drainage indicates failure of conservative management [27].

– Conservative management with dietary control is successful in approximately 50 % of traumatic chylothorax patients [45]. Patients with high output (>1 L/day) are unlikely to respond to conservative management and will require early operative intervention [46].

• Octreotide:

– Octreotide is a somatostatin analogue with a longer half-life, theorised to decreased lymph flow rate, lymph volume, as well as digestive enzyme release and intestinal absorption of fatty acids.
– Prescribed as 50 µg SC/IV q8h
– Initial case series and case reports show some success using octreotide or somatostatin to decrease chyle leak rates however RCTs are lacking [47].

• Surgical Management (TD Ligation):

– Indications:

Failed conservative management
High output leaks (>1 L/day) [45]

– Operative options include: mass ligation of tissue at diaphragmatic hiatus, duct ligation at diaphragmatic hiatus, direct closure of duct injury [27]
– Can be approached via right thoracotomy or right-side VATS
– Olive oil or cream is given PO prior to surgery to improve recognition of duct injury site [27]
– 90 % success rate [45, 48].
– Some surgeons recommend early operative treatment (within 1 week, if patient can tolerate additional surgery) to minimise nutrient loss and immunosuppression from ongoing leak [49–51].

- TD Embolisation (available only in selected centres):
  - TD cannulation rate: 67 %; 90 % resolution of chyle leak post-embolisation [52].
- Prevention:
  - Preoperative oral administration of milk has been shown to facilitate thoracic duct visualisation (95 % vs. 13 %) and decrease risk of duct injury (7 % vs. 13 %) [53].

**Treatment—Non-traumatic Chylothorax**

- Treatment of non-traumatic chylothorax focuses on the treatment of the underlying disease responsible. Concurrent conservative therapy should be instigated (drainage, diet/TPN, +/− octreotide) [54].
- Failure of resolution following treatment of disease requires further intervention [54].
- For malignant chylothorax effusions sclerosant pleurodesis via chest tube or VATS is recommended.
  - Malignant chylothorax patients have limited benefit from TD ligation [55–57].
- For benign or idiopathic chylothorax effusions, thoracoscopic Talc pleurodesis and TD ligation is recommended [45, 58].

# Malignant pleural effusion (MPE)

- Exudative pleural effusion resulting from metastases to pleura
- Approximately 22 % of pleural effusions in the United States; >150,000 cases annually [59]
- Most common causes include metastatic lung, breast, colon and ovarian cancer [19, 60]
- Mean life expectancy of 4–6 months from effusion onset [61, 62]
- Treatment is aimed at palliation of symptoms. Small asymptomatic effusions can be followed [19, 60].

**Therapeutic Thoracocentesis**

- Symptomatic patients can receive serial thoracocentesis, due to the high likelihood of recurrence within weeks following each drainage [19].
- Appropriate for patients with low life expectancy (less than time for recurrence), too frail to receive pleurodesis, or slow pleural effusion recurrence (time to recurrence >1 month) [60].
- Risk of re-expansion pulmonary edema from rapid drainage of large effusions, pneumothorax, and empyema with repeated drainages. Repeated thoracocenteses also produce adhesions which can diminish success of subsequent procedures [62].

**Permanent Indwelling Pleural Catheters (IPC)**

- Indwelling pleural catheter, which patients can drain manually and achieve long-term control.
- Day procedure inserted under local anaesthesia.
- Spontaneous pleurodesis following placement in 40–50 % of patients. When drainage <50 cc/day for 3 days, catheter can be removed [60, 63].
- Indications for catheter placement [60]:
    - Rapid effusion accumulation (<1 month)
    - Life expectancy <3 months
    - Trapped lung
    - Poor operative candidate
    - Failure of chemical pleurodesis
- Contraindications [60]:
    - Slow effusion accumulation (>1 month)
    - Intrapleural adhesions preventing insertion
- Disadvantages: home nursing care of catheter required
- Complications: re-expansion pulmonary edema (patients instructed not to drain >1000 mL/h), catheter malfunction (9.1 %), pneumothorax requiring chest tube (5.9 %), pain (5.6 %), blocked catheter (3.7 %), empyema (2.8 %), cellulitis (3.4 %), IPC fracture during removal [64]

**Pleurodesis**

- Involves initial drainage of effusion, pulmonary re-expansion, and injection of sclerosant into pleural cavity via thoracostomy tube.
- Sclerosants include Talc powder, bleomycin and tetracycline derivatives with success rates of 81–100 %, 61 and 65–76 % respectively using tube thoracostomy instillation [64].
- Local anaesthetics such as lidocaine are often co-injected with sclerosants [65].
- A cost-effective analysis demonstrated chest tube chemical pleurodesis as more cost-effective than IPC placement when patient survival >6 weeks [66].
- Contraindicated in patients who are extremely frail, have an extremely short life expectancy or have trapped lung preventing lung re-expansion (requirement for success of pleurodesis) [19].
- Appropriately selected patients with trapped lung and MPE (a contraindication to simple bed-side pleurodesis) can receive symptomatic benefit from VATS pleurectomy, decortication and pleurodesis [32].
- Cochrane Review Pleurodesis for Malignant Effusions (2004) [67]:

    – Relative Risk (RR) of effusion non-recurrence with sclerosant versus tube thoracostomy drainage alone 1.20 (95 % CI 1.04–1.38) favours using sclerosant [5 studies, 228 subjects].
    – RR of effusion non-recurrence using Talc versus all other sclerosants (tetracycline, bleomycin, mustine and tube thoracostomy drainage alone) 1.34 (95 % CI 1.16–1.55) favours Talc [10 studies, 308 subjects].
    – RR of effusion non-recurrence using thoracoscopic versus bedside tube thoracostomy instillation of Talc 1.19 (95 % CI 1.04–1.36) favours thoracoscopic instillation [2 studies, 112 subjects].
    – RR of effusion non-recurrence using thoracoscopic versus tube thoracostomy bedside instillation of all

sclerosants (Talc, tetracycline, bleomycin, mustine) 1.68 (95 % CI 1.35–2.10) favours thoracoscopic instillation [five studies, 145 subjects].

# General Tube Thoracostomy Pleurodesis Technique (Malignant Effusion)

- *Chest Drainage:*
  - Tube thoracostomy placement, effusion drainage and lung re-expansion
- *Analgesia:*
  - Prior to sclerosant injection intrapleural injection of lidocaine 3 mg/kg (maximum 250 mg) via chest tube is recommended [62]. Alternatively lidocaine may be added to a normal saline Talc solution.
  - Narcotic analgesia is recommended (+/– amnestic agent i.e. midazolam).
- *Sclerosant Options:*
  - *Talc:* 5 g of Talc are dissolved in 100 cc normal saline and placed in two 60 cc Toomey syringes (3 g of Talc are sufficient for pleurodesis for pneumothorax).

    Size-calibrated Talc, <10 % 5–10 μm diameter, is preferred as small particle Talc has been linked to systemic absorption, systemic inflammation and ARDS [68].

  - *Doxycycline:* 500 mg of Doxycycline in 50 cc of normal saline [69]
  - *Bleomycin:* 60 mg of Bleomycin in 50 cc of normal saline [70]
- *Injection of Sclerosant:*
  - Total volume of sclerosant is injected via tube thoracostomy with patient in supine position.
  - Tube thoracostomy is clamped for 1 h.

- Some recommend periodic patient reposition every 15 min (supine, left lateral decubitus, prone, right lateral decubitus) during pleurodesis to allow sclerosant to pool throughout pleural cavity, however this technique is equivalent to patients remaining supine [71].
- After 1 h, the chest tube is placed under −20 cm $H_2O$ wall suction.

- *Drain Removal:*
  - Chest tubes are removed after 24 h or when drainage is <150 cc/day.
  - A randomised trial of 41 patients who received pleurodesis for malignant effusion showed no difference in complications or pleurodesis success between short-term and long-term drainage following pleurodesis [72].

# Tumours of the Pleura: Malignant Pleural Mesothelioma

- Primary tumours of the pleura are very rare. There are two main types:
- *Malignant Pleural Mesothelioma (MM):* most common primary tumour of the pleura. Highly aggressive tumour with grave prognosis.
- *Localised Fibrous Tumour of the Pleura:* significantly less aggressive than MM, also referred to as "localised mesothelioma."

### Epidemiology

- Strong association with asbestos exposure (>80 % of cases), with 20-years latency until the development of MM.
- 5:1 Male predominance, with peak incidence in the sixth-seventh decade.
- Other causes: radiation, mineral fibres, simian virus 40.

## Clinical Presentation

- Dyspnea
- Pain—secondary to chest wall invasion and involvement of somatic nerves of the parietal pleura
- Malignant pleural effusion
- Pleural thickening, subtle pleural masses on radiographic images

  - Thick, restrictive pleural rind (late finding) with encasement of the lung

## Work-Up

- CT chest with IV contrast +/– FDG-PET
- MRI as an adjunct to determine depth of chest wall invasion or diaphragmatic involvement
- Thoracocentesis of malignant effusion: cytology and elevated pleural hyaluronic acid have a 50 % diagnostic accuracy.
- Gold standard for diagnosis is thoracoscopic pleural biopsy.

  - 80 % Diagnostic accuracy

## Management

- Most patients present with locally advanced disease—not amenable to surgical treatment options.
- Surgery is reserved for patients with localised and selected locally advanced disease.

  - Surgery is provided in the context of multi-modality therapy (neoadjuvant or adjuvant chemotherapy and adjuvant whole thorax radiation therapy), with improvement in overall survival and disease-free survival depending on tumour histopathology and regimen.

- *Extrapleural Pneumonectomy (EPP):* en-bloc resection of the lung, visceral pleura, parietal pleura, pericardium, hemidiaphragm.

- Mortality: 0–12 % mortality
- Major perioperative morbidity: 25–55 %
- Low patient compliance with multimodality therapy (50–70 %) [73]
- Provides significant cytoreduction and improved delivery of radiation therapy to target
- Median OS: 13–47 months; DFS: 10–16 months [73]

- *Extended Pleurectomy/Decortication:* less aggressive surgical option than EPP.

  - Mortality: 0–2 %
  - >95 % patient compliance with multimodality therapy [74]

- The optimal surgical option remains controversial. Despite the decrease in cytoreduction compared to EPP, one recent non-randomised trial reports extended pleurectomy/decortication to have improved median survival (23 months vs. 13 months), 2-years survival (49 % vs. 18 %) and 5-years survival (30 % vs. 9 %) [74].
- Whole thorax radiation therapy in conjunction with surgery improves local control.
- Unfortunately, patients with locoregional control from radiotherapy develop systemic disease with limited benefit from chemotherapy (cisplatin/premetrexed: 12-months median survival) [75].
- *Palliative options:* pleurodesis or indwelling pleural catheter drainage to improve quality of life.

# References

1. Noppen M et al. Volume and cellular content of normal pleural fluid in humans examined by pleural lavage. Am J Respir Crit Care Med. 2000;162(3 Pt 1):1023–6.
2. Miserocchi G. Physiology and pathophysiology of pleural fluid turnover. Eur Respir J. 1997;10(1):219–25.
3. Melton 3rd LJ, Hepper NG, Offord KP. Incidence of spontaneous pneumothorax in Olmsted County, Minnesota, 1950 to 1974. Am Rev Respir Dis. 1979;120(6):1379–82.

4. Bense L et al. Nonsmoking, non-alpha 1-antitrypsin deficiency-induced emphysema in nonsmokers with healed spontaneous pneumothorax, identified by computed tomography of the lungs. Chest. 1993;103(2):433–8.

5. Alifano M et al. Atmospheric pressure influences the risk of pneumothorax: beware of the storm! Chest. 2007;131(6):1877–82.

6. Dulchavsky SA et al. Prospective evaluation of thoracic ultrasound in the detection of pneumothorax. J Trauma. 2001;50(2):201–5.

7. Blaivas M, Lyon M, Duggal S. A prospective comparison of supine chest radiography and bedside ultrasound for the diagnosis of traumatic pneumothorax. Acad Emerg Med. 2005;12(9): 844–9.

8. Kelly AM et al. Estimating the rate of re-expansion of spontaneous pneumothorax by a formula derived from computed tomography volumetry studies. Emerg Med J. 2006;23(10):780–2.

9. Baumann MH, Strange C. Treatment of spontaneous pneumothorax: a more aggressive approach? Chest. 1997;112(3): 789–804.

10. Brims FJ, Maskell NA. Ambulatory treatment in the management of pneumothorax: a systematic review of the literature. Thorax. 2013;68(7):664–9.

11. MacDuff A et al. Management of spontaneous pneumothorax: British Thoracic Society Pleural Disease Guideline 2010. Thorax. 2010;65 Suppl 2:ii18–31.

12. O'Rourke JP, Yee ES. Civilian spontaneous pneumothorax. Treatment options and long-term results. Chest. 1989;96(6): 1302–6.

13. Lippert HL et al. Independent risk factors for cumulative recurrence rate after first spontaneous pneumothorax. Eur Respir J. 1991;4(3):324–31.

14. Baumann MH et al. Management of spontaneous pneumothorax: an American College of Chest Physicians Delphi consensus statement. Chest. 2001;119(2):590–602.

15. Naunheim KS et al. Safety and efficacy of video-assisted thoracic surgical techniques for the treatment of spontaneous pneumothorax. J Thorac Cardiovasc Surg. 1995;109(6):1198–203. discussion 1203-4.

16. Heffner JE et al. Clinical efficacy of doxycycline for pleurodesis. Chest. 1994;105(6):1743–7.

17. Kennedy L, Sahn SA. Talc pleurodesis for the treatment of pneumothorax and pleural effusion. Chest. 1994;106(4):1215–22.

18. Thomas R, Lee YC. Causes and management of common benign pleural effusions. Thorac Surg Clin. 2013;23(1):25–42. v-vi.
19. Quinn T et al. Decision making and algorithm for the management of pleural effusions. Thorac Surg Clin. 2013;23(1):11–6. v.
20. Bhatnagar R, Maskell NA. Treatment of complicated pleural effusions in 2013. Clin Chest Med. 2013;34(1):47–62.
21. Aquino SL, Webb WR, Gushiken BJ. Pleural exudates and transudates: diagnosis with contrast-enhanced CT. Radiology. 1994;192(3):803–8.
22. McGrath EE, Anderson PB. Diagnosis of pleural effusion: a systematic approach. Am J Crit Care. 2011;20(2):119–27. quiz 128.
23. Ferrer A et al. Prospective clinical and microbiological study of pleural effusions. Eur J Clin Microbiol Infect Dis. 1999;18(4): 237–41.
24. Menzies SM et al. Blood culture bottle culture of pleural fluid in pleural infection. Thorax. 2011;66(8):658–62.
25. Light RW et al. Pleural effusions: the diagnostic separation of transudates and exudates. Ann Intern Med. 1972;77(4):507–13.
26. Maskell NA, Butland RJ. BTS guidelines for the investigation of a unilateral pleural effusion in adults. Thorax. 2003;58 Suppl 2:ii8–17.
27. Sugarbaker DJ, Lukanich JM. Lung, chest wall, pleura and mediastinum. In: Townsend CM et al., editors. Sabiston textbook of surgery. Philadelphia, PA, USA: Elsevier Inc.; 2012. p. 1564–610.
28. Janda S, Swiston J. Intrapleural fibrinolytic therapy for treatment of adult parapneumonic effusions and empyemas: a systematic review and meta-analysis. Chest. 2012;142(2):401–11.
29. Abu-Daff S et al. Intrapleural fibrinolytic therapy (IPFT) in loculated pleural effusions-analysis of predictors for failure of therapy and bleeding: a cohort study. BMJ Open. 2013;3(2). pii: e001887.
30. Chalmers JD et al. Risk factors for complicated parapneumonic effusion and empyema on presentation to hospital with community-acquired pneumonia. Thorax. 2009;64(7):592–7.
31. MacIver RH. Benign pleural disease. In: Meury CM, Turek JW, editors. TRSA review of cardiothoracic surgery. Chicago, IL, USA: TRSA/TSDA; 2011. p. 54–5.
32. Rathinam S, Waller DA. Pleurectomy decortication in the treatment of the "trapped lung" in benign and malignant pleural effusions. Thorac Surg Clin. 2013;23(1):51–61. vi.
33. Bartlett JG et al. Bacteriology of empyema. Lancet. 1974;1(7853): 338–40.

34. Liu YH et al. Ultrasound-guided pigtail catheters for drainage of various pleural diseases. Am J Emerg Med. 2010;28(8):915–21.
35. Rahman NM et al. The relationship between chest tube size and clinical outcome in pleural infection. Chest. 2010;137(3):536–43.
36. Rahman NM et al. Intrapleural use of tissue plasminogen activator and DNase in pleural infection. N Engl J Med. 2011;365(6): 518–26.
37. Chambers A et al. Is video-assisted thoracoscopic surgical decortication superior to open surgery in the management of adults with primary empyema? Interact Cardiovasc Thorac Surg. 2010; 11(2):171–7.
38. Luh SP et al. Video-assisted thoracoscopic surgery in the treatment of complicated parapneumonic effusions or empyemas: outcome of 234 patients. Chest. 2005;127(4):1427–32.
39. Rahman NM, Kahan BC, Miller RF, Gleeson FV, Nunn AJ, Maskell NA. A clinical score (RAPID) to identify those at risk for poor outcome at presentation in patients with pleural infection. Chest. 2014;145(4):848–55.
40. Valentine VG, Raffin TA. The management of chylothorax. Chest. 1992;102(2):586–91.
41. Franksson C et al. Drainage of thoracic duct lymph in renal transplant patients. Transplantation. 1976;21(2):133–40.
42. Doerr CH et al. Etiology of chylothorax in 203 patients. Mayo Clin Proc. 2005;80(7):867–70.
43. Maldonado F et al. Pleural fluid characteristics of chylothorax. Mayo Clin Proc. 2009;84(2):129–33.
44. Huggins JT. Chylothorax and cholesterol pleural effusion. Semin Respir Crit Care Med. 2010;31(6):743–50.
45. Maldonado F et al. Medical and surgical management of chylothorax and associated outcomes. Am J Med Sci. 2010;339(4): 314–8.
46. Cerfolio RJ et al. Postoperative chylothorax. J Thorac Cardiovasc Surg. 1996;112(5):1361–5. discussion 1365–6.
47. Kalomenidis I. Octreotide and chylothorax. Curr Opin Pulm Med. 2006;12(4):264–7.
48. Paul S et al. Surgical management of chylothorax. Thorac Cardiovasc Surg. 2009;57(4):226–8.
49. Orringer MB, Bluett M, Deeb GM. Aggressive treatment of chylothorax complicating transhiatal esophagectomy without thoracotomy. Surgery. 1988;104(4):720–6.
50. Lagarde SM et al. Incidence and management of chyle leakage after esophagectomy. Ann Thorac Surg. 2005;80(2):449–54.

51. Shirai T, Amano J, Takabe K. Thoracoscopic diagnosis and treatment of chylothorax after pneumonectomy. Ann Thorac Surg. 1991;52(2):306–7.

52. Itkin M et al. Nonoperative thoracic duct embolization for traumatic thoracic duct leak: experience in 109 patients. J Thorac Cardiovasc Surg. 2010;139(3):584–9. discussion 589–90.

53. Shen Y et al. A simple method minimizes chylothorax after minimally invasive esophagectomy. J Am Coll Surg. 2014;218(1): 108–12.

54. McGrath EE, Blades Z, Anderson PB. Chylothorax: aetiology, diagnosis and therapeutic options. Respir Med. 2010;104(1):1–8.

55. Andalib A et al. Influence of postoperative infectious complications on long-term survival of lung cancer patients: a population-based cohort study. J Thorac Oncol. 2013;8(5):554–61.

56. Mares DC, Mathur PN. Medical thoracoscopic talc pleurodesis for chylothorax due to lymphoma: a case series. Chest. 1998; 114(3):731–5.

57. Ferguson MK. Thoracoscopy for empyema, bronchopleural fistula, and chylothorax. Ann Thorac Surg. 1993;56(3):644–5.

58. Graham DD et al. Use of video-assisted thoracic surgery in the treatment of chylothorax. Ann Thorac Surg. 1994;57(6):1507–11. discussion 1511–2.

59. American Thoracic Society. Management of malignant pleural effusions. Am J Respir Crit Care Med. 2000;162(5):1987–2001.

60. Gillen J, Lau C. Permanent indwelling catheters in the management of pleural effusions. Thorac Surg Clin. 2013;23(1):63–71. vi.

61. Burrows CM, Mathews WC, Colt HG. Predicting survival in patients with recurrent symptomatic malignant pleural effusions: an assessment of the prognostic values of physiologic, morphologic, and quality of life measures of extent of disease. Chest. 2000;117(1):73–8.

62. Roberts ME et al. Management of a malignant pleural effusion: British Thoracic Society Pleural Disease Guideline 2010. Thorax. 2010;65 Suppl 2:ii32–40.

63. Light RW. Counterpoint: should thoracoscopic talc pleurodesis be the first choice management for malignant pleural effusion? No Chest. 2012;142(1):17–9. discussion 19–20.

64. Lee P. Point: should thoracoscopic talc pleurodesis be the first choice management for malignant effusion? Yes Chest. 2012;142(1):15–7. discussion 20–1.

65. Feller-Kopman D et al. The relationship of pleural pressure to symptom development during therapeutic thoracentesis. Chest. 2006;129(6):1556–60.

66. Olden AM, Holloway R. Treatment of malignant pleural effusion: PleuRx catheter or talc pleurodesis? A cost-effectiveness analysis. J Palliat Med. 2010;13(1):59–65.
67. Shaw P, Agarwal R. Pleurodesis for malignant pleural effusions. Cochrane Database Syst Rev. 2004;1, CD002916.
68. Gonzalez AV et al. Lung injury following thoracoscopic talc insufflation: experience of a single North American center. Chest. 2010;137(6):1375–81.
69. Putnam Jr JB et al. A randomized comparison of indwelling pleural catheter and doxycycline pleurodesis in the management of malignant pleural effusions. Cancer. 1999;86(10):1992–9.
70. Nikbakhsh N, Pourhasan Amiri A, Hoseinzadeh D. Bleomycin in the treatment of 50 cases with malignant pleural effusion. Caspian J Intern Med. 2011;2(3):274–8.
71. Tan C et al. The evidence on the effectiveness of management for malignant pleural effusion: a systematic review. Eur J Cardiothorac Surg. 2006;29(5):829–38.
72. Goodman A, Davies CW. Efficacy of short-term versus long-term chest tube drainage following talc slurry pleurodesis in patients with malignant pleural effusions: a randomised trial. Lung Cancer. 2006;54(1):51–5.
73. Cao C et al. Systematic review of trimodality therapy for patients with malignant pleural mesothelioma. Ann Cardiothorac Surg. 2012;1(4):428–37.
74. Lang-Lazdunski L et al. Pleurectomy/decortication is superior to extrapleural pneumonectomy in the multimodality management of patients with malignant pleural mesothelioma. J Thorac Oncol. 2012;7(4):737–43.
75. Vogelzang NJ et al. Phase III study of pemetrexed in combination with cisplatin versus cisplatin alone in patients with malignant pleural mesothelioma. J Clin Oncol. 2003;21(14):2636–44.

# Chapter 5
# Mediastinal Disorders

Etienne St-Louis

## Mediastinal Mass: Approach

- The mediastinum can be divided into three compartments (Figs. 5.1 and 5.2). The differential diagnosis (Table 5.1) of a mediastinal mass can therefore be organized according to the compartment in which it is located.
- *Anterior Compartment:* anterior to pericardium and reflection over the great vessels.

  - Includes: thymus gland, lymph nodes, fat
  - In adults, approximately 50 % of mediastinal masses are located in the anterosuperior compartment
  - >90 % consist of thymomas, ectopic thyroid tissue, germ cell tumors, or lymphomas

- *Middle Compartment:* bound by anterior and posterior edges of the pericardium

  - Includes: heart, pericardium, ascending and transverse aorta, brachiocephalic vessels, vena cavae, pulmonary arteries and veins, phrenic and vagus nerves, trachea, bronchi, and lymph nodes

E. St-Louis, M.D., C.M. (✉)
Department of Surgery, McGill University Health Center,
1650 Cedar Avenue, Montreal, QC, Canada H3G 1A4
e-mail: etienne.st-louis@mail.mcgill.ca

A. Madani et al. (eds.), *Pocket Manual of General Thoracic Surgery*, DOI 10.1007/978-3-319-17497-6_5,
© Springer International Publishing Switzerland 2015

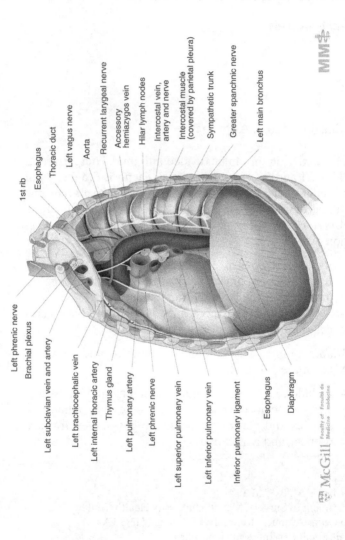

Fig. 5.1. **Medial view of the left hemithorax.** *Used with permission from the McGill University Health Centre Patient Education Office.*

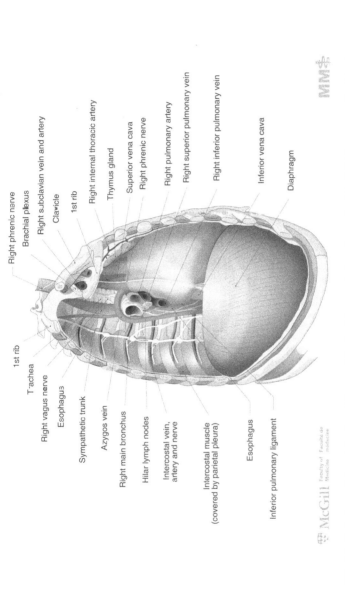

FIG. 5.2. Medial view of the right hemithorax. *Used with permission from the McGill University Health Centre Patient Education Office.*

TABLE 5.1. Differential diagnosis of a mediastinal mass based on compartment.

| Anterosuperior compartment | | Middle compartment | |
|---|---|---|---|
| Thymus | Thymic hyperplasia | Lymph node | *See anterosuperior compartment* |
| | Thymoma | Cyst | Bronchial cyst |
| | Thymic carcinoma | | Pericardial cyst |
| | Carcinoid tumor | | Enteric (duplication) cyst |
| | Small-cell carcinoma | Esophagus | *See posterior compartment* |
| | Thymolipoma | | |

| Posterior compartment | |
|---|---|
| Neurogenic | Schwannoma |
| | Neurofibroma |
| | Ganglioneuroma |
| | Ganglioneuroblastoma |
| | Neuroblastoma |
| Esophagus | Duplication cyst |
| | Diverticulum |
| Other | Benign tumor |
| | Malignant tumor |
| | Meningocele |
| | Paraganglioma |

| Anterosuperior compartment (continued) | |
|---|---|
| Germ cell | Thymic cyst |
| | Teratoma |
| | Dermoid cyst |
| | Seminoma |
| | Choriocarcinoma |
| | Embryonal cell carcinoma |
| | Yolk sac tumor |
| Lymph node | Inflammatory |
| | Infectious |
| | Malignant (metastasis) |
| | Lymphoproliferative disorder (e.g., lymphoma) |
| Mesenchymal | Fibroma/fibrosarcoma |
| | Lipoma/liposarcoma |
| | Lymphangioma |
| | Hemangioma |
| Endocrine | Thyroid |
| | Parathyroid |
| Vascular | Aneurysm |

- *Posterior Compartment:* posterior to pericardium, heart, and trachea and extends to the thoracic vertebral column and paravertebral gutters

  - Includes: esophagus, descending aorta, azygos and hemiazygos veins, thoracic duct, sympathetic chain, and lymph nodes

**Clinical Presentation (Table 5.2):**

- Majority are asymptomatic and discovered incidentally (especially benign lesions)

TABLE 5.2. Clinical presentation of a patient with a mediastinal mass.

| Locoregional symptoms | | Systemic symptoms | |
|---|---|---|---|
| Somatic | Chest pain | Constitutional Symptoms | Night sweats |
| Pulmonary | Cough | | Fatigue |
| | Wheezing | | Weight loss |
| | Stridor | | Pel–Ebstein fevers |
| | Dyspnea | Systemic | Thyrotoxicosis |
| | Hemoptysis | Syndromes | Hypercalcemia |
| | Post-obstructive pneumonitis | | Hypoglycemia |
| | Recurrent pneumonia | | Osteoarthropathy |
| Cardiovascular | Superior vena cava syndrome | | Autoimmune syndrome |
| | Pericardial tamponade | | Paraneoplastic syndrome |
| | Congestive heart failure | | Yolk sac (endodermal cell) tumor |
| Neurogenic | Hoarseness | | |
| | Horner's syndrome | | |
| | Phrenic nerve paralysis | | |
| | Brachial plexopathy | | |

- Symptomatology related to local mass effect, invasion of surrounding structures, and immunologic and hormonal factors related to the lesion. Systemic symptoms (e.g., Type B symptoms) are also seen in lymphoma.
- Physical examination: a full head-to-toe examination, including peripheral lymph nodes and testes in men.
- Diagnosis made by considering the patient's age, location of the mass, presence or absence of locoregional and distant clinical manifestations:

**Workup**

- *Laboratory*: full blood panel, including thyroid function tests, tumor markers (α-fetoprotein (AFP), β-human Chorionic Gonadotropin (βhCG)), cardiac enzymes for chest pain, and autoantibody assays for suspected autoimmune syndromes.
- *Imaging:*
  - Contrast enhanced CT is the modality of choice for detailed characterization of the mass (Fig. 5.3).
  - MRI used as an adjunct to provide additional information about the tissue planes and margins, as well as to differentiate between tumor compression and invasion of surrounding structures.
  - FDG-PET:

    High uptake more likely to correlate with invasiveness and is seen in thymic carcinoma and invasive thymoma [1, 2].
    Comparable sensitivity and specificity to CT scan.
    Significantly higher sensitivity compared with gallium-67 scintigraphy for non-Hodgkin's lymphoma and Hodgkin's lymphoma [3, 4].

- *Tissue diagnosis:*
  - Routine needle biopsy (FNA and core-needle) is typically avoided and the choice of resection or biopsy is made according to the most likely diagnosis based on workup.

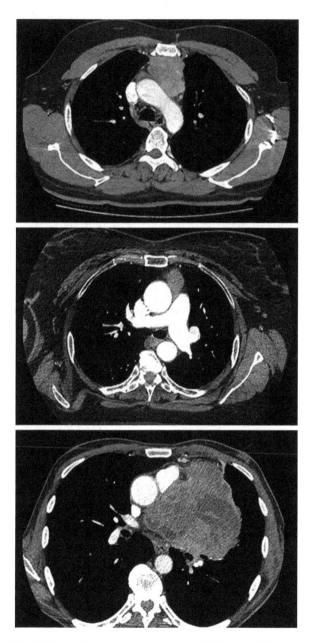

Fig. 5.3. Axial cuts from contrast enhanced CT scan of thymoma in the anterior compartment of the mediastinum.

If lymphoma is suspected, biopsy is required.

Well-encapsulated lesions unlikely to be lymphoma can be directly resected.

Locally invasive and unresectable lesions (other than lymphoma) are typically biopsied and evaluated for possible neoadjuvant therapy (e.g., thymic carcinoma).

- Complications of biopsy include: pneumothorax (20–25 %), hemoptysis (5–10 %), significant hemorrhage (rare), and tumor seeding along needle tract (extremely rare).
- Incisional and excisional biopsies may also be performed under general anesthesia. This may not be possible for patients with high risk of cardiopulmonary compromise (e.g., posture-related dyspnea, SVC syndrome). Options include:

Mediastinoscopic biopsy

2nd/3rd intercostal space parasternal mediastinotomy (Chamberlain procedure)

Transcervical approach

VATS

## Thymoma

### Overview

- Most common neoplasm of the anterosuperior compartment in adults.

  - Incidence: 0.15 per 100,000 person-years in the USA; M = F [5]
  - Rare in the first 2 decades of life
  - Incidence peaks at ages 30–40 (with associated myasthenia gravis (MG)) and 60–70 (without MG) [6]

- Slow-growing epithelial tumor that spreads by local invasion. Extra-thoracic metastases are uncommon [7]

### Pathology

- Controversial distinction between thymomas and thymic carcinomas (Table 5.3).

TABLE 5.3. Classification of mediastinal masses originating from the thymus.

| | |
|---|---|
| Thymus hyperplasia | |
| Epithelial neoplasms | Thymoma |
| | Thymic carcinoma |
| | Thymic neuroendocrine tumors |
| | – Carcinoid tumor |
| | – Small-cell carcinoma |
| Thymolipoma | |
| Thymic cyst | |

- WHO Classification (Table 5.4) stratifies them along a continuum [8].
- Shown to correlate with invasiveness and prognosis [9–11].

**Staging**

- Masaoka clinical staging of thymoma is the most widely used staging system and describes thymomas in terms of local extension of the tumor (Table 5.5).

**Myasthenia Gravis (MG)**

- MG is the most common paraneoplastic syndrome in patients with thymomas (Table 5.6). It is an autoimmune syndrome caused by the production of autoantibodies targeted towards acetylcholine receptors, preventing their activation at the neuromuscular junction.
- Associated with thymus pathology:

  - MG occurs in 20–25 % of patients with thymomas.
  - Thymomas are discovered in 10–20 % of patients with MG.
  - MG in patients with thymomas tends to be more severe and resistant to treatment.

- Manifests as proximal and symmetric muscle weakness (Table 5.7):

  - Ocular (most common): nystagmus, ophthalmoplegia
  - Facial: ptosis, facial droop

TABLE 5.4. WHO classification of thymomas and thymic carcinomas [8].

| WHO classification | Epithelial cell shape | Epithelial cell atypia | Lymphocyte | Organotypic "(Thymus-like)" | Incidence (%) [29] |
|---|---|---|---|---|---|
| A | Spindle | Minimal | Poor | Yes | 9 |
| AB | Spindle/polygonal | Minimal | Moderate | Yes | 24 |
| B1 | Polygonal | Minimal | Abundant | Yes | 13 |
| B2 | Polygonal | Low | Moderate | Yes | 24 |
| B3 | Polygonal | Moderate | Poor | Yes | 15 |
| C (Carcinoma) | | High | Very poor | No | 15 |

Polygonal histologies are divided into B1, B2, B3 according to lymphocyte level, which is also inversely correlated with the level of atypia

TABLE 5.5. Masaoka staging system of thymomas [12].

| Stage | Description |
|---|---|
| I | Macroscopically and microscopically completely encapsulated |
| IIA | Microscopic invasion through capsule |
| IIB | Macroscopic invasion into adjacent fatty tissue or mediastinal pleura |
| IIIA | Macroscopic invasion into adjacent organs (e.g., pericardium or lung) |
| IIIB | Macroscopic invasion of great vessels |
| IVA | Pleural or pericardial dissemination |
| IVB | Lymphogenous or hematogenous metastases |

TABLE 5.6. List of paraneoplastic syndromes in patients with thymomas.

| Paraneoplastic syndrome | |
|---|---|
| Myasthenia gravis | Sjogren syndrome |
| RBC aplasia | Thyroiditis |
| Agammaglobulinemia | Hypercoagulopathy |
| Pure WBC aplasia | Good's syndrome |
| Aplastic anemia | Rheumatoid arthritis |
| Cushing's syndrome | Granulomatous myocarditis |
| Dermatomyositis | Syndrome of inappropriate antidiuretic syndrome |
| Polymyositis | Lambert–Eaton syndrome |
| Progressive systemic sclerosis | |

TABLE 5.7. Osserman–Genkins myasthenia gravis classification [13].

| Grade | Description |
|---|---|
| I | Focal disease (ocular myasthenia) |
| IIA | Mild generalized disease |
| IIB | Moderate generalized disease |
| III | Severe generalized disease |
| IV | Myasthenic crisis with respiratory failure |

- Bulbar: palatal muscle weakness (nasal voice), difficulty chewing, dysphagia, neck extensor weakness
- Limb: dysarthria
- Respiratory (late): diaphragm and intercostal muscle weakness

• Management: acetylcholinesterase inhibitors, steroids, immunomodulators, plasmaphoresis, surgery
• *Surgery:* the benefit of thymectomy in non-thymomatous MG has not been conclusively established [14].

- 35 % of patients with thymomas have complete resolution of MG symptoms after thymectomy, while the majority (60 %) has either a partial improvement in symptoms or remission with medical management [15, 16].

  Very few patients (5 %) have either no change or worsening of symptoms.

- In non-thymomatous MG, up to 50 % resolution and 90 % improvement of symptoms has been reported following thymectomy [17].
- Thymectomy should be offered to all MG patients if no improvement after medical therapies.

**Management**

• Surgery:

- Complete resection is the key to treatment of thymomas and a predictor of survival [11].
- Includes: complete resection of the thymus, all mediastinal tissue anterior to the pericardium, aorta, and SVC, confined by both phrenic nerves laterally, the diaphragm, and the thyroid gland [18].
- Median sternotomy is the most common approach and considered standard of care.
- Other minimally invasive techniques: VATS, transcervical, robotic, and mini-sternotomy approaches.

• *Stage I:* surgery without any neoadjuvant or adjuvant therapy
• *Stages II, III, IVA:* (Fig. 5.4)

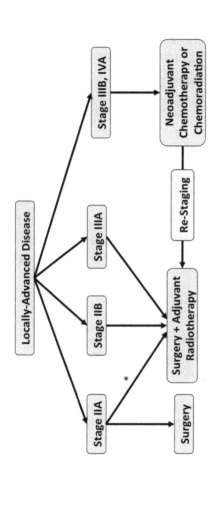

Fig. 5.4. Management algorithm for locally advanced thymomas. *Tumors with high-risk features for recurrence should undergo adjuvant radiotherapy: close margins, high grade, and adherent to adjacent structures.

- The goal of management is complete resection with wide surgical margins.

  - If feasible, surgery should be undertaken. Otherwise, neoadjuvant chemotherapy or chemoradiation can be used to render the tumor resectable.

- Extended resections for locally advanced stage III and IVA disease have shown improved survival [19–21].

  - E.g., pleurectomy, pericardium resection, lung resection, resection of a single phrenic nerve (bilateral resection is not recommended [18]), vascular reconstruction of great vessels

- *Stage IVB:* cisplatin and anthracycline-based chemotherapy is considered first-line therapy [18].
- *Medically unfit for surgery:* chemoradiation or radiation therapy.
- *Unresectable Disease:*

  - For disease that is unresponsive to neoadjuvant therapy, the role of debulking surgery is controversial.

## Thoracic Sympathectomy

### Anatomy and Physiology

- The motor sympathetic route is a chain of three neurons, connecting sudomotor and vasomotor centers, intermediolateral nuclei of spinal gray matter, and paravertebral ganglia to the periphery.
- Only 1 sympathetic paravertebral ganglion per spinal segment.
- *3 Cervical ganglia:*

  - Superior cervical ganglion

    Results from fusion of ganglia of C1-C4, to supply the head and neck.
    Located at level of transverse process of C2-C3.

– Middle cervical ganglion

Results from fusion of ganglia of C5-C6.
Located at level of transverse process of C6.

– Cervicothoracic (stellate) ganglion

Results from fusion of the inferior most cervical gan-
glion (C7) and the first thoracic ganglion.
Located anterior to the head of the first rib.
Denervation results in Horner syndrome.

• *Thoracic ganglia:*

– Positioned anterior to transverse processes of thoracic
vertebrae and covered by parietal pleura.
– Fewer ganglia than thoracic spinal segments due to
fusion of the first thoracic ganglion with C7 ganglion,
fusion of ganglia of T12 with L1 and fusion of thoracic
ganglia with each other.
– Greater and lesser splanchnic nerves originate from
preganglionic fibers of T5-T12 and innervate the
medulla of the adrenal glands.

• Sympathetic adrenergic fibers innervate blood vessel
smooth muscles.

– Vasomotor tone depends only on sympathetic vasocon-
strictor fibers.
– Greatest effect on arterioles (influence on skin circulation > great vessels and muscular arteries).

• Sympathetic cholinergic fibers innervate apocrine sweat
glands.

– Different neural centers control various types of sweating
through reflex pathways.

Emotion sweating—Cortical
Thermal sweating—Hypothalamic
Gustatory sweating—Medullary

**Indications for Thoracic Sympathectomy**

- *Idiopathic Hyperhidrosis:*

  - Production of excess quantities of sweat due to central stimulation of the sympathetic system.
  - Prevalence = 3–5 % [22]
  - Most intense during adolescence (rarely begins in childhood, and may persist into adulthood) [23].
  - Palmar hyperhidrosis has the greatest clinical significance due to social and professional implications.
  - Moderate hyperhidrosis may be amenable to topical agents, systemic medical therapy (anticholinergic agents), iontophoresis, or Botulinum toxin injections with limited efficacy.
  - Severe hyperhidrosis and cases refractory to other forms of therapy can undergo surgery with >95 % success rate [24].

- *Thromboangiitis obliterans:*

  - Vaso-occlusive disease, with unknown etiology leading to inflammatory changes in small and medium sized arteries and veins causing pain, ischemia, and gangrene.
  - Management: smoking cessation, avoidance of vasoconstrictive stimuli, pain control, supportive care, and surgery as a last resort.

- *Complex regional pain syndrome:*

  - Regional pain conditions often occur after injury with disproportionate response to the inciting event.
  - Management: multimodality therapy

    Physical therapy and psychotherapy
    Pharmacologic therapy: NSAIDs, corticosteroids, antidepressants, sympatholytics
    Nonsurgical interventions: peridural/intrathecal infusions, spinal cord stimulation
    Chemical or surgical sympathectomy: weak evidence to support this option—mostly anecdotal [25]

- *Long QT syndrome:*

  - Idiopathic congenital disorder characterized by lengthened QT segment on EKG associated with high incidence of severe tachyarrhythmia and sudden cardiac death. Untreated mortality rate: 75–80 %.
  - Severe episodes occur during intense physical exercise or emotional crises suggesting potential role for sympathectomy.
  - While beta blockers are effective in preventing 80 % of crises, sympathectomy is potentially indicated for the remaining 20 % with ongoing syncopal episodes despite appropriate medical treatment [26].

- *Raynaud Phenomenon:*

  - Idiopathic episodes of arteriolar spasm in digits, most common in young women and precipitated by exposure to cold, emotional upset, or drugs.
  - During crises, patients complain of pain, hypothermia, numbness, and paresthesia.

    If frequent, this may result in subsequent ischemic lesions in affected fingers.

  - Despite the limited evidence for thoracic sympathectomy, 95 % of patients show improvement in ulcer healing [27].

**Surgical Approach**

- VATS considered standard of care for thoracic sympathectomy.

  - The thoracic sympathetic chain is identified through the pleura as a white, multinodular cord forming a slight prominence in the posterolateral region of the vertebrae, above the heads of costal arches.
  - The target ganglion varies depending on the therapeutic intent of surgery (Table 5.8).

TABLE 5.8. Target ganglia based on the therapeutic intent for a thoracic sympathectomy.

| Disease | Denervation level |
| --- | --- |
| Palmar hyperhidrosis | T3-T4 |
| Axillary hyperhidrosis | T4 |
| Craniofacial hyperhidrosis | T2 |
| Facial rubor | T2 |
| Complex regional pain syndrome | Stellate, T2, T3 |

- Complications (15 %) [28]:

  - Compensatory sweating (10 %)

    Generalized reflex increase in sweating post-sympathectomy.

    Incidence varies depending on the level and extent of sympathectomy (lowest rates occur with single ganglion blockade and denervation at T3 and T4).

  - Pneumothorax (1.5 %)
  - Segmental atelectasis
  - Rare: Horner's syndrome, hyperhidrosis recurrence, gustatory sweating, hemothorax, chylothorax, arrhythmia

# References

1. Kumar A, et al. Characterization of thymic masses using (18) F-FDG PET-CT. Ann Nucl Med. 2009;23(6):569–77.
2. Lococo F, et al. Role of combined 18F-FDG-PET/CT for predicting the WHO malignancy grade of thymic epithelial tumors: a multicenter analysis. Lung Cancer. 2013;82(2):245–51.
3. Kostakoglu L, et al. Comparison of fluorine-18 fluorodeoxyglucose positron emission tomography and Ga-67 scintigraphy in evaluation of lymphoma. Cancer. 2002;94(4):879–88.
4. Wirth A, et al. Fluorine-18 fluorodeoxyglucose positron emission tomography, gallium-67 scintigraphy, and conventional staging for Hodgkin's disease and non-Hodgkin's lymphoma. Am J Med. 2002;112(4):262–8.
5. Engels EA, Pfeiffer RM. Malignant thymoma in the United States: demographic patterns in incidence and associations with subsequent malignancies. Int J Cancer. 2003;105(4):546–51.

6. Detterbeck FC, Parsons AM. Thymic tumors. Ann Thorac Surg. 2004;77(5):1860–9.
7. Regnard JF, et al. Prognostic factors and long-term results after thymoma resection: a series of 307 patients. J Thorac Cardiovasc Surg. 1996;112(2):376–84.
8. Müller-Hermelink HK, Krenning EP, Kuo TT, et al. Tumours of the thymus. In: Travis WD, Brambilla E, Muller-Hermelink HK, Harris CC, editors. World Health Organization Classification of tumours. Pathology and genetics of tumours of the lung, pleura, thymus and heart. Lyon, France: IARC Press; 2004. p. 148–51.
9. Kim DJ, et al. Prognostic and clinical relevance of the World Health Organization schema for the classification of thymic epithelial tumors: a clinicopathologic study of 108 patients and literature review. Chest. 2005;127(3):755–61.
10. Kondo K, et al. WHO histologic classification is a prognostic indicator in thymoma. Ann Thorac Surg. 2004;77(4):1183–8.
11. Okumura M, et al. Clinical and pathological aspects of thymic epithelial tumors. Gen Thorac Cardiovasc Surg. 2008;56(1):10–6.
12. Masaoka A, et al. Follow-up study of thymomas with special reference to their clinical stages. Cancer. 1981;48(11):2485–92.
13. Osserman KE, Genkins G. Studies in myasthenia gravis: review of a twenty-year experience in over 1200 patients. Mt Sinai J Med. 1971;38(6):497–537.
14. Cea G, et al. Thymectomy for non-thymomatous myasthenia gravis. Cochrane Database Syst Rev. 2013;10, CD008111.
15. Okumura M, et al. Biological implications of thymectomy for myasthenia gravis. Surg Today. 2010;40(2):102–7.
16. Lucchi M, et al. Association of thymoma and myasthenia gravis: oncological and neurological results of the surgical treatment. Eur J Cardiothorac Surg. 2009;35(5):812–6. discussion 816.
17. Gronseth GS, Barohn RJ. Thymectomy for myasthenia gravis. Curr Treat Options Neurol. 2002;4(3):203–9.
18. Falkson CB, et al. The management of thymoma: a systematic review and practice guideline. J Thorac Oncol. 2009;4(7):911–9.
19. Moore KH, et al. Thymoma: trends over time. Ann Thorac Surg. 2001;72(1):203–7.
20. Sugiura H, et al. Long-term results of surgical treatment for invasive thymoma. Anticancer Res. 1999;19(2B):1433–7.
21. Yagi K, et al. Surgical treatment for invasive thymoma, especially when the superior vena cava is invaded. Ann Thorac Surg. 1996;61(2):521–4.

22. Adar R, et al. Palmar hyperhidrosis and its surgical treatment: a report of 100 cases. Ann Surg. 1977;186(1):34–41.
23. Strutton DR, et al. US prevalence of hyperhidrosis and impact on individuals with axillary hyperhidrosis: results from a national survey. J Am Acad Dermatol. 2004;51(2):241–8.
24. Drott C, Gothberg G, Claes G. Endoscopic transthoracic sympathectomy: an efficient and safe method for the treatment of hyperhidrosis. J Am Acad Dermatol. 1995;33(1):78–81.
25. Straube S, et al. Cervico-thoracic or lumbar sympathectomy for neuropathic pain and complex regional pain syndrome. Cochrane Database Syst Rev. 2013;9, CD002918.
26. Schwartz PJ, et al. Left cardiac sympathetic denervation in the therapy of congenital long QT syndrome. A worldwide report. Circulation. 1991;84(2):503–11.
27. Coveliers HM, et al. Thoracic sympathectomy for digital ischemia: a summary of evidence. J Vasc Surg. 2011;54(1):273–7.
28. Oncel M, et al. Bilateral thoracoscopic sympathectomy for primary hyperhydrosis: a review of 335 cases. Cardiovasc J Afr. 2013;24(4):137–40.
29. Detterbeck FC. Clinical value of the WHO classification system of thymoma. Ann Thorac Surg. 2006;81(6):2328–34.

# Chapter 6
## Chest Wall Disorders

**Amin Madani**

## Congenital Disorders

- Rare conditions with highly variable clinical presentations anywhere from asymptomatic to severe physiologic effects secondary to poor respiratory mechanics and lung development.

### Pectus Excavatum

- Central depression of the chest secondary to posterior angulation of the sternum and costal cartilages.

    - Symmetric or asymmetric with a greater frequency of right-sided depression.
    - May worsen throughout the rapid growth of adolescence.

- Most common congenital chest wall deformity; associated with Marfan's syndrome [1], scoliosis (26 %) [2] and congenital heart disease (1.5 %) [3].

A. Madani, M.D. (✉)
Department of Surgery, McGill University,
Montreal, QC, Canada
e-mail: amin.madani@mail.mcgill.ca

A. Madani et al. (eds.), *Pocket Manual of General
Thoracic Surgery*, DOI 10.1007/978-3-319-17497-6_6,
© Springer International Publishing Switzerland 2015

- *Physiologic consequences:*

  - Can result in reduced lung volumes and capacities on spirometry.
  - Pressure on the right ventricle and annulus may lead to reduced cardiac output and mitral valve prolapse.

- *Clinical Presentation*:

  - Mostly asymptomatic
  - Reduced exercise tolerance
  - Pain (uncommon)
  - Psychological effects due to aesthetic concerns of the patient
  - *Haller index* used to measure the degree of deformity [4].

    Transverse chest diameter divided by the anterior–posterior diameter on CT (Fig. 6.1).

- *Management*: surgery (gold standard).

  - Aim: produce superior cosmetic results with alleviation of the physiologic effects.
  - Indications: severe, progressive or symptomatic disease, compromised pulmonary physiology, Haller index >3.25 and compression on the heart impairing cardiac function [5]
  - Ravitch repair—open repair:

    Resection of abnormal costal cartilages
    Correcting the posterior displacement of the sternum

  - Nuss procedure—minimally invasive technique using thoracoscopy to guide the retrosternal placement of a stainless steel bar that remains in place for 2–3 years (Fig. 6.2).

    Preferred method over open repair
    Complications (<5 %): bar displacement, bar allergy, pneumothorax requiring thoracostomy tube, and unsatisfactory cosmetic result. Very uncommon complications include cardiac injury and erosion into the sternum.

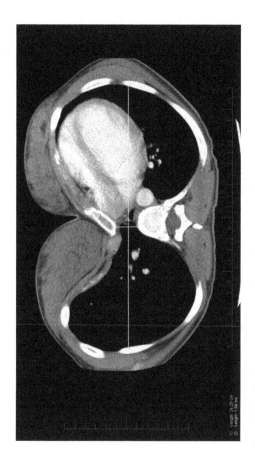

FIG. 6.1. The Haller index is the transverse chest diameter divided by the anterior–posterior diameter on CT. This patient had a Haller index of 12 before undergoing surgery.

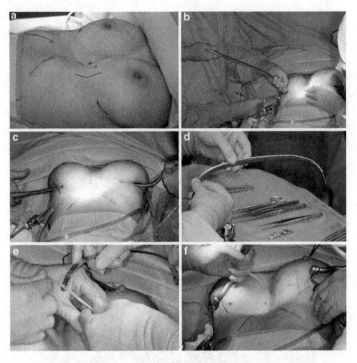

Fig. 6.2. The Nuss procedure involves thoracosopic insertion of a steel bar retrosternally. (**a**) This patient had Pectus Excavatum (Haller index 12). (**b**, **c**) under thoracoscopic guidance, an insertion device is channelled underneath the sternum. (**d**–**f**) the bar (implant) is shaped intraoperatively according to the patient's chest wall and passed through that same tract using an umbilical tape.

Both techniques have shown to improve pulmonary function tests (forced expiratory volume in 1 s, forced vital capacity, vital capacity, total lung capacity) after 1 year, with a greater improvement using the Nuss technique following bar removal [6].

**Pectus Carinatum**

- Anterior protrusion of the sternum
- Unlike Pectus Excavatum, it is more likely to present in later childhood and with pain.

- Surgical repair involves subperichondrial resection of the costal cartilages involved with sternum osteotomy depending on the type of deformity.
- Some success reported using orthotic bracing in younger children, despite poor compliance.

***Sternal Defects*: Deformities occurring as a result of the failure of fusion of the sternum during development**

- *Sternal Cleft:*

    - Normal overlying skin, with normal heart position
    - Repaired in early infancy using direct closure

- *Ectopia Cordis ("Herniated Heart"):*

    - Heart protrudes anteriorly without any overlying tissue
    - *Cervical Ectopia Cordis: s*ignificant protrusion of the heart, occasionally fused to the head

- *Cantrell's Pentalogy (Thoracoabdominal Ectopia Cordis):*

    - Sternal cleft, diaphragmatic defect (absence of septum transversum), pericardial defect, epigastric omphalocele and cardiac anomaly. The heart is covered by a thin membrane and often displaced into the abdomen through the diaphragmatic defect.

**Poland's Syndrome**

- Hypoplasia of the pectoralis major and minor, associated with syndactyly or brachydactyly

    - Mostly unilateral, with occasional involvement of the breast (amastia and athelia)
    - Increased rates of childhood leukaemia [7]

- Surgical repair is indicated when there is underlying chest wall deformity leading to functional deficit.

TABLE 6.1.  Chest wall tumour: differential diagnosis.

| Primary | Benign | Malignant |
|---|---|---|
| Bone | Ostoblastoma | Ewing sarcoma[a] (8–22 %) |
| | Osteoid osteoma | Osteosarcoma[a] (10 %) |
| Cartilage | Chondroma[a] | Chondrosarcoma[a] (20 %) |
| | Osteochondroma[a] | |
| Fibrous tissue | Fibrous dysplasia[a] | Fibrosarcoma |
| | Desmoid tumour[a] (fibroma) | |
| Vascular | Hemangioma | Hemangiosarcoma |
| Adipose tissue | Lipoma | Liposarcoma |
| Muscle | Leiomyoma | Leiomyosarcoma |
| | Rhabdomyoma | Rhabdomysarcoma |
| Nerve | Neurofibroma | Neurofibrosarcoma |
| | Schwannoma | Malignant schwannoma |
| | | Neuroblastoma |
| Miscellaneous | | Solitary plasmacytoma[a] (10–30 %) |
| | | Lymphoma[a] (Hodgkin, non-Hodgkin) |
| | | Leukaemia |
| Secondary | Metastasis or local invasion from adjacent organs: | |
| | Breast, melanoma, lung, thyroid, mesothelioma, renal cell | |

[a]Most common

# Primary Chest Wall Tumours

- Rare and highly heterogeneous group of tumours (Table 6.1).
- Over 60 % are malignant, with a higher rate of malignancy in young children and the elderly [8–10].

## Clinical Presentation

- Majority present with a palpable (60 %), enlarging, hard and painful mass; minority (<30 %) are asymptomatic, most of which are benign [9].

  - Pain (40 %) occurs as a results of periosteal or neural invasion.

- Growth rate is dependent on tumour type.
- Metastasis or local invasion from a secondary lesion are more common and should be ruled out.

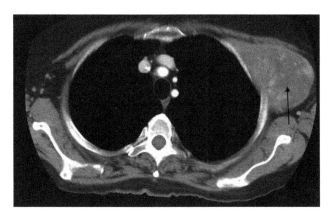

Fɪɢ. 6.3. CT image of a chest wall tumour (*black arrow*).

**Workup**

- Imaging: MRI, CT, PET-CT

  - CT with IV contrast provides considerable detail regarding size, location, local invasion, involvement of other structures, and metastatic spread (Fig. 6.3).
  - MRI provides better resolution, anatomic delineation of the tissue planes and characterization of soft-tissue masses.

    Mostly performed for tumours in the thoracic inlet and extremities.

  - PET-CT provides additional accuracy for diagnosis and staging, but its role has yet to be established.

- Tissue diagnosis will allow for appropriate staging of the primary tumour and subsequent management. This is normally done using either core needle biopsy or excisional biopsy. Incisional biopsies can be performed for larger tumours, without compromising subsequent resection.

**Management**

- The majority of tumours with no metastasis are treated with wide resection with or without reconstruction.

  - The role of chemotherapy or radiotherapy is highly dependent on the specific histopathology.

- Outcomes after surgical resection show a 1-, 5- and 10-year survival of 90, 60 and 50 %, respectively [10].

  - Recurrence occurs in 50 %, with a 5-year survival of 17 %, depending on the primary tumour [10].

- *Benign tumours:*

  - The majority are treated with wide-resection.
  - *Desmoid tumours:* locally aggressive and invasive with a high recurrence rate (25–75 %) [11, 12].

    Positive margins have a 90 % 5-year probability of developing recurrence compared to 18 % with negative margins [13].

    Radiation therapy can also be given in the adjuvant setting for patients with positive margins, when surgery is contraindicated, or for large bulky tumours.

- *Chondrosarcoma:*

  - The majority (80 %) originate from the ribs and can be related to prior trauma to the chest wall.
  - Highly resistant to chemoradiation; surgical resection is the preferred treatment.

- *Solitary Plasmacytoma:*

  - This aggressive form of multiple myeloma has a high propensity to spread systemically.
  - After workup and exclusion of extra-thoracic disease, the lesion is treated with radiation therapy, with or without surgical resection.

- *Ewing sarcoma:*

  - Aggressive, occurring commonly in young males; may also present with constitutional symptoms.

- Managed using multimodality therapy; mostly with neoadjuvant chemotherapy followed by surgical resection. Radiation therapy may also be used in the adjuvant setting.

- *Osteosarcoma:*
  - Treated with neoadjuvant chemotherapy followed by surgical resection.
  - Tumour response to chemotherapy and presence of metastasis predict prognosis [8, 14].

- *Soft-tissue sarcoma:*
  - Consist of 6 % of all soft tissue sarcomas and 45 % of chest wall tumours [8].
  - Treated with wide resection.
  - Radiation therapy given as neoadjuvant treatment for large tumours >5 cm, as adjuvant therapy for residual disease, or for instances when wide resection is done with <1 cm margins.

**Principles of Surgical Resection and Reconstruction**

- When indicated, wide resection for malignant and aggressive benign tumours should be performed with a 4 cm circumferential margin, although this margin size is controversial and dependent on the tumour type.

  - Bone invasion requires entire bone removal, along with any other structures involved.

- *Goals of resection*: to provide an oncologically sound resection, while maintaining adequate pulmonary function and providing stability and integrity to the chest wall.
- With large defects, reconstruction may be required.

  - Primary closure is generally satisfactory for resection of one rib or less, defects <5 cm, and certain posterior lesions <10 cm that are covered by the scapula (provided there is no risk for entrapment of the tip of the scapula).
  - Reconstruction is typically required for all other defects.

- *Reconstruction technique options*:

  - Autologous tissue using pedicled flaps:

    Muscle flap with either primary skin closure or skin graft. Options include latissimus dorsi, rectus abdominis, pectoralis major, external oblique and serratus anterior muscles.

    Myocutaneous flap—either free or pedicled.

  - Prosthesis:

    Non-rigid meshes—Gore-Tex, PTFE, Marlex, Prolene, Vicryl.

    Rigid prosthesis—methyl methacrylate, sternum/rib fixation.

  - Considerable controversy exists with regard to the optimal reconstruction technique.

    Despite higher complication rates, rigid fixation has been advocated as the preferred method to provide stability for the chest wall, preventing flail segments and subsequent respiratory insufficiency [15]. Nonetheless, it can be complicated by prosthesis infection, pain and chest wall deformities.

    A recent study using myocutaneous pedicled flaps with or without non-rigid prosthesis reported a 5 % surgical site infection rate (compared to 7–20 % for rigid fixation in historical cohorts), including no infections occurring after 30 days and only 3 % reoperation for infected meshes (compared to 8–12 % for rigid fixation) [16–19]. Despite a slightly higher rate of pneumonia in this cohort, hospital stay was significantly shorter, and long-term follow-up revealed no chronic pain or cosmetic deformities.

  - *Complications:*

    Respiratory complications can be caused by altered pulmonary physiology. These include issues with oxygenation (atelectasis, pneumonia or ARDS) or distorted chest wall mechanics (poor cough, flail segment), all of which can lead to respiratory failure and severe morbidity.

Surgical-site infections may require re-operation and mesh explantation.

- *Follow-up:* serial CT scans for local recurrence or distant metastasis (pulmonary and hepatic).

# Thoracic Outlet Syndrome (TOS)

### Pathophysiology

- Thoracic outlet is a compact anatomical space bordered by the middle scalene muscle posteriorly, the clavicle superiorly and the first rib inferiorly (Fig. 6.4).
- As the brachial plexus, subclavian artery and subclavian vein travel through the thoracic outlet to the upper limb, they may be subject to external compression from a variety of causes, including cervical rib, anterior scalene hypertrophy, costoclavicular syndrome or trauma, leading to a constellation of symptoms known as TOS.

### Clinical Presentation: various forms of TOS occur depending on the aetiology, either individually or in combination

- *Neurogenic TOS (90 %):* limb pain, numbness, tingling or weakness most commonly in the dominant arm

  – There is no gold standard for diagnosis.

- *Venous TOS (5 %):* pain, swelling or cyanotic discoloration of the limb

  – *Paget–Schroetter Syndrome* occurs when venous TOS leads to thrombosis of the axillary or subclavian vein after repetitive motion.

- *Arterial TOS (1–5 %):* arm fatigue with or without ischaemic changes in the digits

  – Caused by repetitive local trauma and arterial wall injury, which may lead to stenosis, aneurysm formation, distal embolization and ischaemia [20–22].

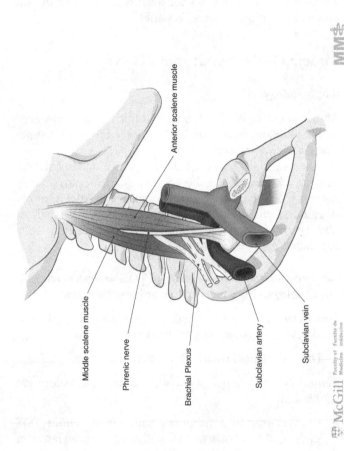

FIG. 6.4. Thoracic outlet anatomy. *Used with permission from the McGill University Health Centre Patient Education Office.*

- Physical examination includes a full musculoskeletal and neurovascular assessment of both affected and non-affected limbs, with the addition of the following manoeuvres despite their low specificity and sensitivity:

  - Adson manoeuvre: with the patient's head turned towards the contralateral side, the radial pulse disappears during deep breaths due to arterial compression.
  - Upper limb tension test: the patient is asked to open and close their hand repeatedly for 3 min, while abducting the arm >90° with external rotation. This will elicit pain in neurogenic TOS.

**Workup**

- While CT scan with IV contrast can delineate vascular structures, MRI provides better resolution of soft-tissue abnormalities.
- X-rays can be done to rule out a cervical rib or other vertebral anomaly that may cause compression of the underlying structures.
- Contrast arteriogram and venogram can also be done if there is a high suspicion for arterial or venous TOS.
- All images should be obtained in both a neutral position and other positions, where the patient's arm is positioned in a location that will reproduce compression of the affected structure(s).
- There is no gold standard for the diagnosis of neurogenic TOS.

**Management**

- Neurogenic TOS is initially managed with a trial of physical rehabilitation for several months.

  - Refractory cases (over 50 %) should be referred for surgical intervention [23].

- Arterial TOS is more urgent and should be treated surgically.

  - Decompression is usually done via either a transaxillary or supraclavicular approach, with the latter becoming increasingly more popular.
  - The artery is generally bypassed and any structures that are compressing the thoracic outlet are resected (the first rib is normally removed and anterior and middle scalenectomies are performed).
  - If distal embolization has occurred, the patient should undergo either thrombolysis or embolectomy [20].

- Venous TOS is treated with thrombolysis and subsequent surgical decompression.
- Complications: injury to the phrenic nerve, branches of the brachial plexus, or thoracic duct, and pneumothorax if the pleural cavity has been entered.
- Immediate post-operative rehabilitation should follow to maintain range-of-motion and function of the affected limb [23, 24].

# References

1. Scherer LR, et al. Surgical management of children and young adults with Marfan syndrome and pectus excavatum. J Pediatr Surg. 1988;23(12):1169–72.
2. Waters P, et al. Scoliosis in children with pectus excavatum and pectus carinatum. J Pediatr Orthop. 1989;9(5):551–6.
3. Shamberger RC, Welch KJ. Cardiopulmonary function in pectus excavatum. Surg Gynecol Obstet. 1988;166(4):383–91.
4. Haller Jr JA, Kramer SS, Lietman SA. Use of CT scans in selection of patients for pectus excavatum surgery: a preliminary report. J Pediatr Surg. 1987;22(10):904–6.
5. Kelly Jr RE. Pectus excavatum: historical background, clinical picture, preoperative evaluation and criteria for operation. Semin Pediatr Surg. 2008;17(3):181–93.

6. Chen Z, et al. Comparative pulmonary functional recovery after Nuss and Ravitch procedures for pectus excavatum repair: a meta-analysis. J Cardiothorac Surg. 2012;7:101.

7. Boaz D, Mace JW, Gotlin RW. Poland's syndrome and leukaemia. Lancet. 1971;1(7694):349–50.

8. Burt M. Primary malignant tumors of the chest wall. The Memorial Sloan-Kettering Cancer Center experience. Chest Surg Clin N Am. 1994;4(1):137–54.

9. Hsu PK, et al. Management of primary chest wall tumors: 14 years' clinical experience. J Chin Med Assoc. 2006;69(8):377–82.

10. King RM, et al. Primary chest wall tumors: factors affecting survival. Ann Thorac Surg. 1986;41(6):597–601.

11. Allen PJ, Shriver CD. Desmoid tumors of the chest wall. Semin Thorac Cardiovasc Surg. 1999;11(3):264–9.

12. Kabiri EH, et al. Desmoid tumors of the chest wall. Eur J Cardiothorac Surg. 2001;19(5):580–3.

13. Abbas AE, et al. Chest-wall desmoid tumors: results of surgical intervention. Ann Thorac Surg. 2004;78(4):1219–23. discussion 1219–23.

14. Bieling P, et al. Tumor size and prognosis in aggressively treated osteosarcoma. J Clin Oncol. 1996;14(3):848–58.

15. Smith SE, Keshavjee S. Primary chest wall tumors. Thorac Surg Clin. 2010;20(4):495–507.

16. Hanna WC, et al. Reconstruction after major chest wall resection: can rigid fixation be avoided? Surgery. 2011;150(4):590–7.

17. Lardinois D, et al. Functional assessment of chest wall integrity after methylmethacrylate reconstruction. Ann Thorac Surg. 2000;69(3):919–23.

18. Chang RR, et al. Reconstruction of complex oncologic chest wall defects: a 10-year experience. Ann Plast Surg. 2004;52(5):471–9. discussion 479.

19. Losken A, et al. A reconstructive algorithm for plastic surgery following extensive chest wall resection. Br J Plast Surg. 2004; 57(4):295–302.

20. Marine L, et al. Arterial thoracic outlet syndrome: a 32-year experience. Ann Vasc Surg. 2013;27(8):1007–13.

21. Sanders RJ, Hammond SL, Rao NM. Diagnosis of thoracic outlet syndrome. J Vasc Surg. 2007;46(3):601–4.

22. Patton GM. Arterial thoracic outlet syndrome. Hand Clin. 2004;20(1):107–11. viii.

23. Thompson RW, Petrinec D. Surgical treatment of thoracic outlet compression syndromes: diagnostic considerations and transaxillary first rib resection. Ann Vasc Surg. 1997;11(3):315–23.
24. Thompson RW, Petrinec D, Toursarkissian B. Surgical treatment of thoracic outlet compression syndromes. II. Supraclavicular exploration and vascular reconstruction. Ann Vasc Surg. 1997;11(4):442–51.

# Chapter 7
## Chest Trauma

**Ali Aboalsaud and Dan L. Deckelbaum**

## Pneumothorax

**Pathophysiology**

- Abnormal presence of air within the pleural cavity.
- Lung compression reduces lung compliance, volumes, and diffusion capacity.
- **Tension Pneumothorax:**
  - If left untreated, air can accumulate without decompressing adequately, leading to high positive pleural pressures, causing severe lung collapse, and compression of the mediastinum, great vessels, and heart, and ultimately hemodynamic compromise secondary to decreased venous return.
  - Patients in tension pneumothorax require immediate needle decompression in the second intercostal space at the mid-clavicular line, followed by tube thoracostomy.

**Mechanism**

- Abnormal communication between the pleural cavity and either the alveoli or airways cause the air to flow into the

A. Aboalsaud, M.D. (✉) • D.L. Deckelbaum
Department of Surgery, McGill University Health Center,
Montreal, QC, Canada
e-mail: ali.aboalsaud@gmail.com

A. Madani et al. (eds.), *Pocket Manual of General Thoracic Surgery*, DOI 10.1007/978-3-319-17497-6_7,
© Springer International Publishing Switzerland 2015

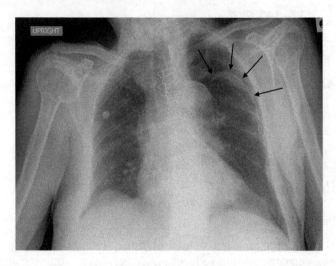

FIG. 7.1. Patient presenting with a traumatic pneumothorax after blunt trauma to the chest. *Black arrows* denote the outline of the collapsed lung.

pleural cavity, eliminating its negative pressure and leading to collapse of the lung (Fig. 7.1). This can happen with penetrating or blunt chest traumas.

- Massive air leak suggests injury to major airways.
- Penetrating: Air enters the pleural cavity either directly through the wound in the chest wall or from a parenchymal laceration caused by the injury.
- Blunt: Parenchymal laceration secondary to an associated injury (rib fracture, bronchial rupture, alveolar rupture).
- **Open Pneumothorax (Sucking Chest Wound):**
  - Air enters the pleural cavity through the chest wall defect with inspiration, thereby eliminating the pressure gradient between the pleural cavity and alveoli.
  - Should be initially covered with a 3-way occlusive dressing, followed by tube thoracostomy and an occlusive dressing.

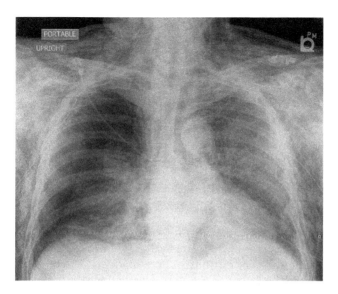

Fɪɢ. 7.2. Significant subcutaneous emphysema seen on the chest X-ray of a patient with a pneumothorax after blunt trauma to the chest.

**Diagnosis**

- Pleuritic chest pain and dyspnea are the most common symptoms.
- On primary survey, several signs are indicative of a pneumothorax, including decreased or absent breath sounds, subcutaneous emphysema (Fig. 7.2), and hyperresonance. A tension pneumothorax may also present with tracheal deviation to the contralateral side, severe respiratory distress, and hemodynamic instability.
- Diagnosis is established by an upright chest X-ray. If clinical signs of tension physiology are evident, X-ray confirmation should be omitted and immediate decompression should ensue, followed by a chest tube.

  - An expiratory view accentuates the separation of the parietal and visceral pleura.

- Pneumothorax in supine patients accumulates into the dependent regions of the anterior and subdiaphragmatic pleura and may be detected as a deep sulcus sign.
- CT scan is the gold standard for diagnosis and can detect occult pneumothoraces undetected by chest radiograph.
- Ultrasound is also an accurate, rapid, and noninvasive test in trauma patients.

  Sensitivity: 95–98 %; true-negative rate: 100 % [1, 2]
  Subcutaneous emphysema can interfere significantly with ultrasound.

**Management**

- Management depends on the clinical setting, mechanism of injury, size of the pneumothorax, and associated conditions. Advanced Trauma Life Support (ATLS) guidelines should be followed for all trauma patients [3].
- The appropriate initial diagnostic tests and management options should be tailored to the presentation of the patient:

  - Hemodynamically unstable patients with clinical signs of a pneumothorax should have a large-bore chest tube placed as part of the primary survey (with or without needle decompression preceding it for suspected tension pneumothorax).
  - For patients who are stable, imaging studies can confirm the diagnosis prior to definitive management.

- *Observation:*

  - Reserved for asymptomatic patients with small or occult pneumothoraces who are unlikely to have an ongoing air leak. Follow-up radiography should be obtained at 3 h to document improvement or to make sure there is no worsening.
  - Supplemental oxygen can help decrease the concentration of nitrogen in the body, thus creating a gradient to drive the air in the pleura (mostly composed of nitrogen) into the body.

- *Percutaneous Catheters:*
  - Small- to medium-calibre tube thoracostomy can be performed percutaneously via the Seldinger technique and attached to either a Heimlich one-way valve or a suction.
  - Use is limited to a pneumothorax with small or no associated hemothorax.

- *Tube Thoracostomy:*
  - Large-bore chest tubes are the standard of care for treatment of traumatic pneumothoraces, unstable patients, persistent or large air leaks, and associated effusions or hemothoraces.

# Hemothorax

### Mechanism and Pathophysiology

- Abnormal presence of blood in the pleural cavity.
- Significant hemothorax may be caused by injury to the great vessels, heart, lung parenchyma, or chest wall/intercostal vessels, secondary to either blunt or penetrating injury.

### Diagnosis

- Clinical presentation and diagnosis are similar to pneumothorax, except for dullness to percussion.
- Upright chest X-ray will confirm the diagnosis if >300 mL of blood is present (Fig. 7.3).
- Hemodynamically unstable patients with signs of pneumo-hemothorax require immediate decompression without imaging.

### Management

- ATLS protocols should be followed, starting with a primary and secondary survey.
- Goal is complete removal of all blood. Residual blood is a nidus for the development of empyema and fibrothorax,

---

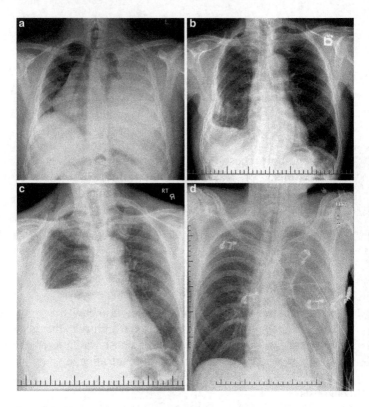

FIG. 7.3. Traumatic hemothorax diagnosed on chest X-ray. (**a**) Patient presenting with a massive left hemothorax after blunt trauma to the chest. The mediastinal structures, including the heart, trachea, and major airways, are shifted to the right. Typically blood can be identified on upright chest X-ray (**b**, **c**); however this may not always be the case if the patient is supine (**d**).

which can also occur due to improper positioning or obstruction of the chest tube [4].

– If this is not feasible with one chest tube, residual blood can either be removed by additional chest tube(s) or surgically (thoracoscopically if patient is clinically stable).

- Posttraumatic empyema can also occur secondary to a foreign body, lung abscess, bronchopleural fistula, esophageal perforation, or an abdominal source [5]. *See* Chap. 4: *Pleural Disorders (Empyema).*
- Tube thoracostomy is initially performed using a 32–36 French chest tube.
- Indications for thoracotomy:
  - Hemodynamic instability
  - >1,500 mL of blood drains initially upon insertion of chest tube
  - Persistent bleeding of >200 mL/h for 4 h

# Chest Wall Injuries

- The types of chest wall injuries vary depending on the mechanism of trauma, force of injury, and the patient's characteristics. Certain injuries such as fractures of the first rib, sternum, scapula, lower ribs, and bilateral ribs are associated with other life-threatening injuries.

## *Rib Fractures:*

### Mechanism and Pathophysiology:

- Most common injury following blunt chest trauma (30–40 % of all thoracic trauma) [6].
- Physiologic sequelae of rib fractures are related to their impact on normal pulmonary mechanics mostly due to significant pain, causing decreased ability to cough, reduced lung volumes, and an increased risk for pneumonia.

  - This is especially true for the elderly who have reduced chest wall compliance, reduced bone density, and higher incidence of underlying lung disease [7].

- *Flail Chest:* Occurs when three or more adjacent ribs are fractured in two places (Fig. 7.4). The most common mechanism is direct-impact injury (e.g., steering wheel).

  - Leads to severe disruption of lung mechanics with paradoxical motion during breathing, placing patients at very high risk of respiratory failure. Patients also often have severe pulmonary contusions.
  - Paradoxical motion may not be obvious during positive-pressure ventilation.

**Management**

- Aggressive pain control is fundamental in managing rib fractures and improving lung mechanics. For limited rib fractures (≤3) in healthy young adults, this might be the only necessary management and can be carried out as an outpatient.

  - Various methods available: regional anaesthesia, epidural infusion, paravertebral block, intrapleural infusion, patient-controlled analgesia pumps, oral or intravenous narcotics, and nonsteroidal anti-inflammatories.

- Chest physiotherapy, incentive spirometry, and frequent pulmonary toilet should be encouraged.
- Patients with severe respiratory compromise may require mechanical ventilation.
- Surgical fixation (Fig. 7.5) is indicated in select patients [8]. Acceptable indications include:

  - Flail chest
  - Pain refractory to conservative management options
  - Significant chest wall deformity
  - Chest wall instability and symptomatic nonunion
  - Displaced ribs found on thoracotomy performed for other reasons
  - Open fractures

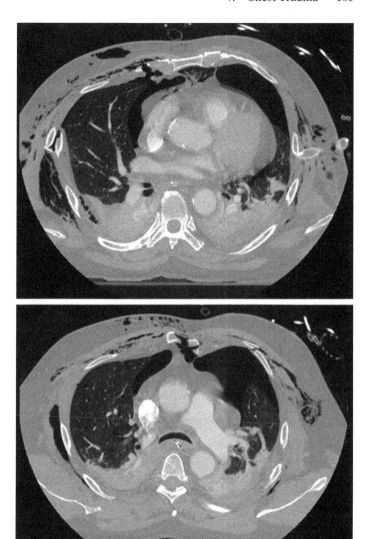

FIG. 7.4. Patient presenting with multiple rib fractures, sternal fracture, flail chest, and associated lung injuries (bilateral pneumohemothoraces and pulmonary contusions) after a crush injury to the chest. Subcutaneous emphysema can be seen throughout the anterior and lateral chest wall.

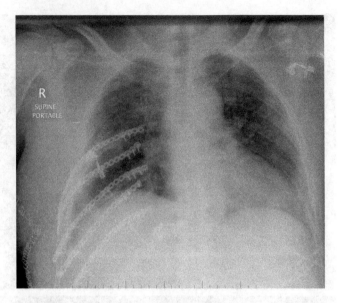

Fig. 7.5. Patient with flail chest who underwent surgical fixation.

## *Sternal Fracture:*

**Mechanism**

- Occurs in less than 0.5 % of all traumas [9].
- Most commonly caused after rapid deceleration from motor vehicle collisions.
- Almost always transverse at the sternomanubrial joint or midbody of the sternum.
- Associated with the use of three-point restraints.
- Can be associated with other injuries due to the large force necessary required to cause fracture—especially in unrestrained passengers and crush injuries.

- Associated injuries include rib fractures, myocardial contusion, vertebral fractures, hemopericardium, hemothorax, pneumothorax, and retrosternal hematoma.

- Patients should undergo a CT scan to rule out other injuries and an electrocardiogram to screen for blunt cardiac injury (BCI) (Fig. 7.4).

**Management**

- Initially, care is directed towards the primary and secondary survey, exclusion of other injuries, and adequate pain control.
- According to the severity of the fracture and associated injuries, the patient might need a surgical fixation (if severely displaced or unstable fractures) or cardiac monitoring [10, 11].

# Pulmonary Contusions

**Mechanism and Pathophysiology:**

- Bruising of the lung, mostly caused by blunt thoracic trauma and associated with chest wall injuries.
- Blood accumulating in the alveoli results in right-to-left shunting, leading to ventilation-perfusion mismatch and subsequent hypoxia.
- Radiographic evidence of contusions may be delayed, and appear only 24–48 h after the injury (Fig. 7.6).

**Management**

- Pulmonary contusions are managed similarly to all chest wall injuries, including treating associated injuries, pain control, pulmonary toilet, incentive spirometry, and chest physiotherapy.

  - Excessive volume resuscitation can exacerbate the negative physiologic consequences of pulmonary contusions.
  - Aim is to maintain euvolemia.

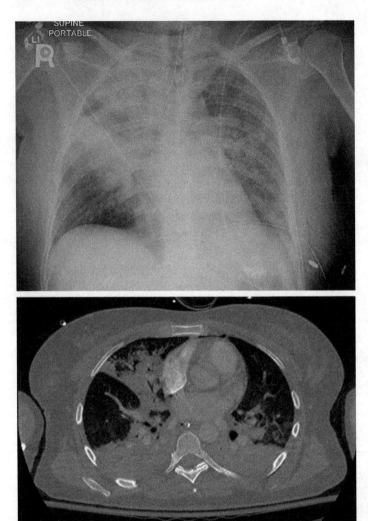

FIG. 7.6. Bilateral pulmonary contusions after blunt trauma to the chest.

# Blunt Cardiac Injury

## Mechanism and Pathophysiology

- The incidence of BCI after blunt thoracic injury is approximately 20 %, occurring most commonly with motor vehicle collisions [14].
- BCI can manifest itself in several forms, ranging from minor electrocardiogram changes to heart failure and septal or free wall rupture.
- The most common BCIs are myocardial contusion (60–100 %), right ventricular injury (17–32 %), and right atrial injury (8–65 %) [14].

## Diagnosis

- Electrocardiogram is the initial investigation of choice.
- Any arrhythmias (e.g., sinus tachycardia, nonspecific ST or T wave changes, heart block, or other forms of dysrhythmias) should be followed by a transthoracic echocardiogram.
- Controversy exists regarding the utility of troponin levels for patients suspected of having BCI, and given the lack of evidence to support its use, many experts recommend against it. However, the latest Eastern Association for the Surgery of Trauma (EAST) guidelines have changed and now recommend both electrocardiogram and troponin I level for all patients suspected to have suffered BCI (negative predictive value: 100 %) [15].

**Management: See Fig. 7.7**

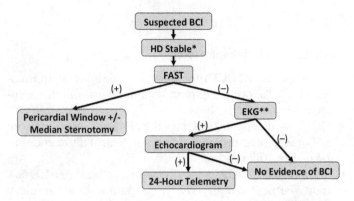

FIG. 7.7. Management algorithm for blunt cardiac injury (BCI). *EKG* electrocardiogram, *HD* hemodynamically. *Hemodynamically unstable patients are managed separately based on ATLS management protocols.* **Some experts also recommend ordering troponin I levels to screen for BCI.*

## Diaphragmatic Injuries

### Mechanism

- More common after penetrating (4 %) than blunt (1 %) thoracoabdominal trauma [16].
- *Penetrating:* Direct injury to the diaphragm
- *Blunt*: Sudden increase in intra-abdominal pressure
- Blunt diaphragmatic injuries are more common on the left due to the liver's absorptive capacity protecting the right hemidiaphragm.

### Diagnosis

- Early diagnosis can avoid herniation and possibly strangulation of intra-abdominal content into the chest.

- In patients with other indications for surgical intervention, injury to the diaphragm is ruled out intraoperatively either through the abdomen (laparotomy or laparoscopy) or the thorax (thoracotomy or VATS).
- For patients without any other indications for surgical intervention, diagnosis may be difficult.
- Chest X-ray can demonstrate herniated viscus in the thorax (unless positive-pressure ventilation prevents this), and other signs that are suggestive of injury, such as lower rib and sternal fractures, an elevated hemidiaphragm (Fig. 7.8), and a nasogastric tube traveling back up into the

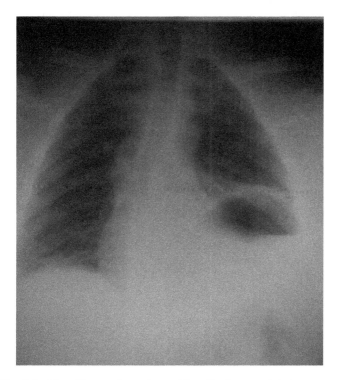

FIG. 7.8. Chest X-ray of a patient with a diaphragmatic injury.

chest. Sensitivity however is limited using this and other imaging modalities (i.e., CT, FAST).

- Hemodynamically stable patients who have clinical suspicion of a diaphragmatic injury should be evaluated by either laparoscopy (preferred) or thoracoscopy. If laparoscopy is used, it should be performed after other intra-abdominal injuries have been ruled out.

**Management**

- All patients already undergoing trauma laparotomy or thoracotomy for other reasons should undergo careful examination of the diaphragm (Fig. 7.9).
- Most diaphragmatic injuries should be repaired with non-absorbable sutures, usually via the abdomen due to the high likelihood of associated injuries [17]. Select hemodynamically stable patients who would otherwise not be explored surgically, with an asymptomatic, small, right-sided injury that is tamponaded by the liver, may be observed.

# Approach to Penetrating Chest Trauma Management (Fig. 7.10)

### Resuscitative, Emergency Department (ED) Thoracotomy

- ED thoracotomy is a life-saving procedure that is performed for patients with specific injuries who have had a recently witnessed loss of measurable blood pressure or palpable pulse (Table 7.1).

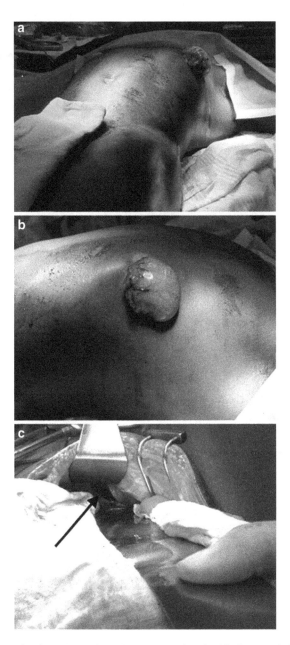

FIG. 7.9. (**a-c**) Patient with a left penetrating (stab) thoracoabdominal injury with the stomach is seen herniating through the chest. This patient underwent an exploratory laparotomy and the diaphragmatic defect (*black arrow*) was identified and repaired. *Used with permission from Dr. Dan L Deckelbaum.*

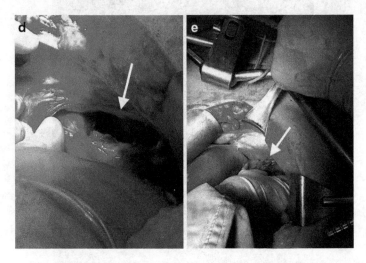

Fig. 7.9. (continued) (**d-e**) Another patient with a similar left diaphragmatic injury (*white arrow*) that was repaired after an exploratory laparotomy using non-absorbable sutures.

- Outcomes vary significantly amongst patients, with survival rates of 3–35 % in isolated cardiac injuries, 1–14 % in penetrating trauma, and 0–1 % in blunt trauma [12].
- The ED thoracotomy is limited to very few life-saving therapeutic maneuvers (Fig. 7.11):

  - Releasing a pericardial tamponade
  - Open cardiac massage
  - Cross-clamping the descending aorta
  - Controlling hemorrhage (cardiac or other intrathoracic sources)

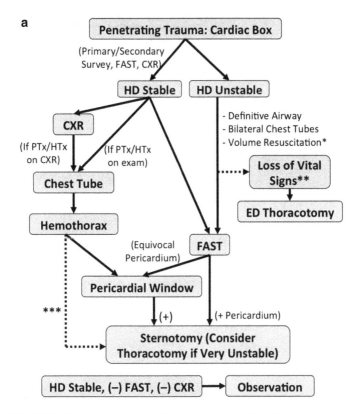

FIG. 7.10. Management algorithms for penetrating chest trauma to the cardiac box (**a**) and lateral/posterior chest (**b**). *HD* hemodynamic, *CXR* chest X-ray, *FAST* Focused Assessment for the Sonographic evaluation of Trauma, *PTx* pneumothorax, *HTx* hemothorax, *ED* emergency department. *Volume resuscitation includes placing large-bore peripheral or central venous catheters and massive transfusion protocol. **Criteria for resuscitative thoracotomy should be met prior to its initiation. ***Significant hemothorax should be followed by a thoracotomy (i.e., >1,500 mL, or >200 mL/h × 4 h).

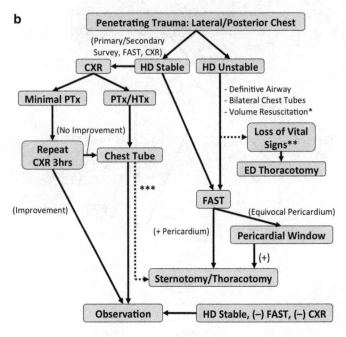

FIG. 7.10. (continued)

TABLE 7.1. Indications for a resuscitative thoracotomy [13].

Penetrating trauma
-   Loss of vital signs in the ED
-   Loss of vital signs <15 min prior to arrival

Blunt trauma
-   Loss of vital signs in the ED
-   Loss of vital signs <5 min prior to arrival

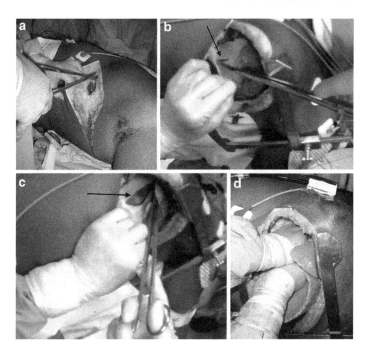

FIG. 7.11. An ED thoracotomy performed on a patient with a penetrating trauma to the chest. After making the incision just below the nipple line (**a**) and getting access to the chest cavity, a pericardiotomy is performed (*black arrow*) to decompress any potential cardiac tamponade (**b, c**). Cardiac massage (**d**) can also be performed using a two-hand technique. *Used with permission from Dr. Dan L Deckelbaum.*

# References

1. Dulchavsky SA et al. Prospective evaluation of thoracic ultrasound in the detection of pneumothorax. J Trauma. 2001;50(2):201–5.
2. Blaivas M, Lyon M, Duggal S. A prospective comparison of supine chest radiography and bedside ultrasound for the diagnosis of traumatic pneumothorax. Acad Emerg Med. 2005;12(9):844–9.

3. Advanced trauma life support for doctors student course manual. 8th ed. American college of Surgeons Committee on Trauma. 2008.
4. Aguilar MM et al. Posttraumatic empyema. Risk factor analysis. Arch Surg. 1997;132(6):647–50. discussion 650–1.
5. Mandal AK et al. Posttraumatic empyema thoracis: a 24-year experience at a major trauma center. J Trauma. 1997;43(5):764–71.
6. Sirmali M et al. A comprehensive analysis of traumatic rib fractures: morbidity, mortality and management. Eur J Cardiothorac Surg. 2003;24(1):133–8.
7. Bergeron E et al. Elderly trauma patients with rib fractures are at greater risk of death and pneumonia. J Trauma. 2003; 54(3):478–85.
8. Lafferty PM et al. Operative treatment of chest wall injuries: indications, technique, and outcomes. J Bone Joint Surg Am. 2011;93(1):97–110.
9. Recinos G et al. Epidemiology of sternal fractures. Am Surg. 2009;75(5):401–4.
10. von Garrel T et al. The sternal fracture: radiographic analysis of 200 fractures with special reference to concomitant injuries. J Trauma. 2004;57(4):837–44.
11. Peek GJ, Firmin RK. Isolated sternal fracture: an audit of 10 years' experience. Injury. 1995;26(6):385–8.
12. Rhee PM et al. Survival after emergency department thoracotomy: review of published data from the past 25 years. J Am Coll Surg. 2000;190(3):288–98.
13. Moore EE et al. Defining the limits of resuscitative emergency department thoracotomy: a contemporary Western Trauma Association perspective. J Trauma. 2011;70(2):334–9.
14. Schultz JM, Trunkey DD. Blunt cardiac injury. Crit Care Clin. 2004;20(1):57–70.
15. Clancy K et al. Screening for blunt cardiac injury: an Eastern Association for the Surgery of Trauma practice management guideline. J Trauma Acute Care Surg. 2012;73(5 Suppl 4):S301–6.
16. Rubikas R. Diaphragmatic injuries. Eur J Cardiothorac Surg. 2001;20(1):53–7.
17. Hanna WC, Ferri LE. Acute traumatic diaphragmatic injury. Thorac Surg Clin. 2009;19(4):485–9.

# Chapter 8
# Benign Esophageal Disorders

**Maria Abou-Khalil and Amin Madani**

## Esophagus: Anatomy and Physiology

### Anatomy (Table 8.1; Fig. 8.1)

### Physiology

Swallowing: Oropharyngeal Phase (1.5 s)

1. Elevation of tongue—bolus pushed into posterior oropharynx (voluntary)
2. Posterior movement of tongue—bolus pushed into hypopharynx (voluntary)
3. Elevation of soft palate—close off passage into nasopharynx
4. Elevation of hyoid—brings epiglottis under tongue
5. Elevation of larynx—opens retrolaryngeal space
6. Tilting of epiglottis—covers opening of larynx

M. Abou-Khalil
Department of Surgery, McGill University Health Center,
Montreal, QC, Canada

A. Madani, M.D. (✉)
Department of Surgery, McGill University,
Montreal, QC, Canada
e-mail: amin.madani@mail.mcgill.ca

A. Madani et al. (eds.), *Pocket Manual of General Thoracic Surgery*, DOI 10.1007/978-3-319-17497-6_8,
© Springer International Publishing Switzerland 2015

TABLE 8.1. Vasculature, lymphatics, and innervation of the esophagus.

| | Cervical esophagus | Thoracic esophagus | Abdominal esophagus |
|---|---|---|---|
| Arterial supply (segmental) | • Inferior thyroid artery<br>• Superior thyroid artery (cricopharyngeus muscle) | • Aorta (4–6 esophageal branches)<br>• Left/right bronchial arteries (esophageal branches)<br>• Branches of: inferior thyroid, intercostal, inferior phrenic arteries | • Left gastric artery<br>• Inferior phrenic arteries |
| | • All arterial branches terminate in a capillary network forming rich collaterals outside and within the submucosa, along the entire length of the esophagus<br>→ Allows the esophagus to be surgical mobilized with a low risk of ischemia | | |
| Venous supply (segmental) | • Inferior thyroid veins | • Venae comitantes (surround esophagus)<br>→ Azygos, hemiazygos veins | • Inferior phrenic veins<br>• Left gastric vein (coronary vein), short gastric veins |
| | • First basin of venous drainage is the rich submucosal venous plexus which drains into the superficial periesophageal venous plexus<br>→ Allows for very rapid spread of infection and tumor to three body cavities | | |

| | | |
|---|---|---|
| Lymphatic drainage (non-segmental) | • Paratracheal nodes<br>• Deep cervical, internal jugular nodes | • Superior and posterior mediastinal nodes (paratracheal, subcarinal, paraesophageal, retrocardiac, infracardiac, para-aortic, inferior pulmonary ligament nodes) | • Gastric and celiac nodes |

• Extensive lymphatic networks in the lamina propria, submucosa, muscularis propria, and adventitia → Allows for very rapid spread of infection and tumor to three body cavities
• Very extensive longitudinal and transmural drainage—unpredictable lymphatic spread

| | | |
|---|---|---|
| Innervation | • Vagus nerve: Recurrent and superior laryngeal nerve<br>• Cervical sympathetic trunk | • Vagus nerve: Direct branches<br>• Thoracic sympathetic trunk | • Vagus nerve: Anterior/posterior plexus<br>• Greater and lesser splanchnic nerves |

• Vagus nerve provides motor, sensory, parasympathetic, and sympathetic innervation
• Injury to the RLN can lead to dysmotility, hoarseness, and aspiration
• Intrinsic innervation: Myenteric (Auerbach) plexus and submucosal (Meissner) plexus

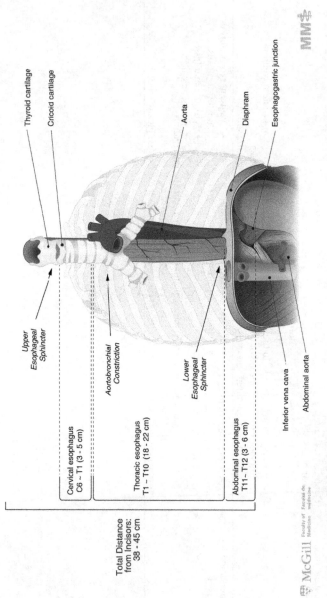

Fig. 8.1. Esophageal anatomy. *Used with permission from the McGill University Health Centre Patient Education Office.*

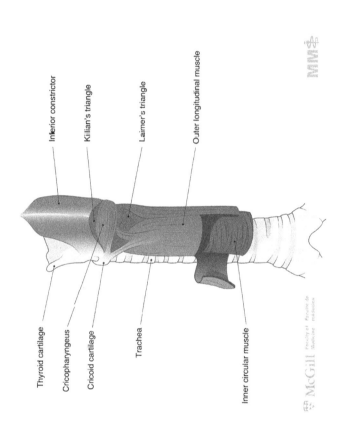

Thyroid cartilage

Cricopharyngeus

Cricoid cartilage

Trachea

Inner circular muscle

Inferior constrictor

Killian's triangle

Laimer's triangle

Outer longitudinal muscle

McGill Faculty of Medicine / Faculté de médecine

FIG. 8.1. (continued)

## Swallowing: Esophageal Phase

### Upper Esophageal Sphincter

- High-pressure region between pharynx and esophagus, tonically contracted at 60 mmHg (2–3 cm length) via the cricopharyngeus muscle to prevent reflux and aspiration
- During swallowing, upper esophageal sphincter (UES) relaxes, while posterior pharyngeal constrictors propel food boluses into the esophagus using a pressure differential between the cervical esophagus (positive pressure) and intrathoracic esophagus pressures (negative pressure)
- UES subsequently closes, reaching 90 mmHg pressure for 2–5 milliseconds, marking the start of peristalsis
- UES relaxes back to its resting tonic pressure of 60 mmHg

### Peristalsis

- Primary

  - Progressive contractions, moving down the esophagus at 2–4 cm/s
  - Reaches LES 9 s after initiation of voluntary swallowing
  - Intraluminal pressure: 40–80 mmHg

- Secondary

  - Progressive contractions initiated by distension or irritation of esophagus (not voluntary swallowing)
  - Clears esophagus of leftover food from primary peristalsis

- Tertiary

  - Uncoordinated, nonprogressive contractions
  - Responsible for esophageal spasm

### Lower Esophageal Sphincter

- Not a true sphincter; corresponds only to a slight thickening of the esophageal muscularis layer
- High-pressure zone 2–5 cm in length, resting tonic pressure 6–26 mmHg (minimum 1 cm intra-abdominal for normal

lower esophageal sphincter (LES) function) as barrier to reflux
- Respiratory inversion point (RIP): Transition from intra-thoracic to intra-abdominal LES
- Transient relaxation of 5 s, occurring 2–3 s after oropharyngeal phase

# Gastroesophageal Reflux Disease

## Pathophysiology

- Abnormal flow of gastric content into the esophagus, secondary to abnormalities of:
  - LES
  - Esophageal peristalsis
  - Hiatal hernia affecting competency of GEJ

- Mucosal injury leads to pain, cough, heartburn, dysphagia, and regurgitation
- Complications: Esophagitis (Fig. 8.2), strictures, extraesophageal symptoms (laryngopharyngeal reflux disease), metaplastic or neoplastic changes (*See* Chap. 9: *Esophagus*: *Malignant Disorders*)

## Management: Nonsurgical

- Lifestyle interventions: weight loss, elevation of the head of the bed, avoidance of meals before bedtime, avoidance of foods that decrease LES tone
- Medical:
  - Antacids (calcium carbonate, sodium bicarbonate, aluminum and magnesium hydroxide):

    Provide rapid short-term relief, but limited role for the treatment of erosive esophagitis

  - Histamine 2 receptor antagonists:

    Can heal mild esophagitis, or adjunct to proton-pump inhibitors (PPI) for acid breakthrough

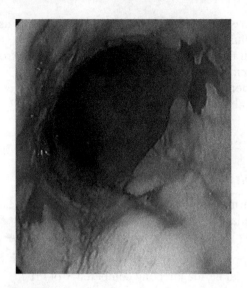

FIG. 8.2. Esophagitis.

- PPI (mainstay of treatment):

  Superior healing rates and decreased relapse rates for erosive esophagitis and non-erosive reflux disease compared to other medical therapy

- Prokinetic agents (domperidone, metoclopramide):

  Useful in patients with delayed emptying and gastroparesis

- Sucralfate:

  Binds to mucosa, preventing injury

- GABA-B agonist (baclofen):

  Use is very limited due to side-effect profile on the central nervous system

## Management: Antireflux Surgery

- Antireflux surgery (ARS) is more effective than medical management for treating gastroesophageal reflux disease (GERD) [1].

- However, given the efficacy of medical management and its limited side-effect profile, first-line treatment for GERD is PPI with lifestyle modifications.

- Indications of ARS
  - Failed medical management
  - Patients who cannot take long-term PPIs (e.g., cost, compliance, side effects)
  - Patients with respiratory symptoms or vocal cord damage secondary to reflux
- Although many patients have regression of metaplasia (Barrett's esophagus), it is generally not performed as a cancer-prevention strategy [2].
- Objective evidence of GERD is required prior to proceeding with ARS—e.g., 24-h pH monitoring or reflux esophagitis on endoscopy.
- Goal of ARS is to restore a competent LES.
- Options: Laparoscopic fundoplication

  - Nissen: 360° wrap posteriorly (complete wrap)
  - Toupet: 270° posteriorly (partial wrap)
  - Dor: 180° anteriorly (partial wrap)
  - Hill: 180° posteriorly (partial wrap)—rarely performed due to anchoring to preaortic fascia and the risk of vascular injury

- Partial wraps have decreased postoperative dysphagia compared to Nissen fundoplication and thought to be a better option for patients with motility disorders (e.g., achalasia)—however this is controversial.
- No difference in postoperative reflux recurrence between partial and complete wraps [3, 4].
- Technical elements:

  - Division of short gastric vessels
  - Extensive posterior mediastinal dissection (mobilize GEJ >2 cm intra-abdominally)
  - Closure of crura using a bougie
  - Securing fundoplication (gastropexy)

- Treatment of GERD in the context of morbid obesity is best managed with bariatric procedures.

# Paraesophageal Hernia

## Hiatal Hernia (HH) Classification (Fig. 8.3)

1. Type I (Sliding HH): most common (>95 %); intra-abdominal GEJ → intrathoracic
2. Type II paraesophageal hernia (PEH): Least common; GEJ at its normal anatomical location, but an enlarged esophageal hiatus allowing the stomach fundus to herniate into the thoracic cavity
3. Type III PEH: Combination of Type I and II, with displaced GEJ and stomach herniation through the hiatus
4. Type IV PEH: Herniation of other intra-abdominal organs into the thoracic cavity (spleen, colon, omentum, etc.)

## Pathophysiology

- Increased age: Loss of elasticity and weakening of the phreno-esophageal ligament
- Increased intra-abdominal pressure (due to obesity, ascites, chronic cough, pregnancy)

## Gastric Volvulus

- Stomach most common organ to herniate and is occasionally associated with gastric volvulus

### Organoaxial volvulus

- Stomach rotated around the axis from the phrenoesophageal membrane to the pylorus
- Antrum rotates creating an "upside-down stomach"
- 60 % of all gastric volvulus
- Associated with PEH and high rates of strangulation and necrosis (5–28 %)

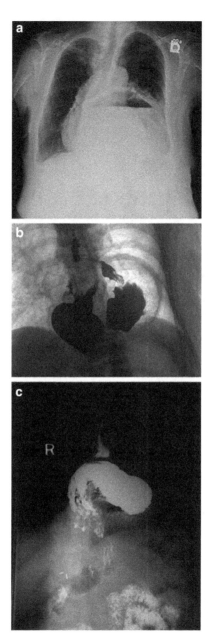

FIG. 8.3. Chest X-ray (**a**) and upper GI contrast studies (**b**, **c**) of Type III paraesophageal hernias.

**Mesoenteroaxial volvulus**

– Stomach rotation around axis which bisects greater and lesser curve
– Posterior stomach becomes anterior
– Not always associated with PEH

## Clinical Presentation

- Intermittent solid food dysphagia (acute obstruction)
- Intermittent and postprandial epigastric or chest pain (50 %)

    – Acute severe pain: Need to rule out gastric volvulus and strangulation

- Heartburn and/or regurgitation (30–50 %) [5, 6]
- GI bleeding from gastric ischemia → mucosa ulceration (Cameron's ulcer); chronic iron-deficiency anemia

**Strangulation**

– Severe and persistent pain, +/– fever, retching without vomiting

## Evaluation

- Esophagogram:

    – Diagnosis and anatomical delineation of stomach relative to diaphragm
    – Rule out volvulus or strangulation

- Esophagogastroscopy:

    – Direct evaluation of gastric mucosa during strangulation
    – Rule out other pathology

- Manometry and 24-h pH studies are of limited use in large hiatal hernias
- CT scan (particularly coronal images)

## Management (Fig. 8.4)

*Approach:* **Laparoscopic/transabdominal, thoracoscopic/transthoracic**

- Similar recurrence rates; shorter length of stay, lower morbidity and pain using laparoscopy
- Laparoscopic PEH repair is currently the standard of care for all primary hiatal hernias. Open transthoracic approaches may have a role in recurrent cases.

### Principles of PEH repair

1. Hernia reduction
2. Hernia sac dissection +/– resection
3. Hernia defect closure
4. Antireflux procedure to prevent high rates of postoperative reflux
5. GEJ restoration to normal anatomic location

### Strangulation

- Immediately decompress stomach with nasogastric tube
- Surgical emergency: Necrosis, perforation → mediastinitis; 50–80 % mortality

  - Viable stomach: Repair PEH with fundoplication

    Although feasible via laparoscopic approach, the strangulated PEH may require open repair to reduce the stomach delicately if the gastric wall is edematous/inflamed.

  - Nonviable stomach (Fig. 8.5): Partial vs. total gastrectomy, depending on the degree of necrosis

    Typically, the fundus is the only necrotic component, thereby sparing the lesser curvature and allowing for a sleeve gastrectomy

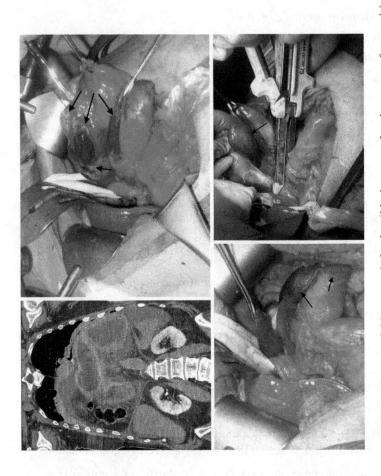

Fig. 8.4. Strangulated PEH with a nonviable stomach fundus (*black arrows* showing areas of necrosis). This patient

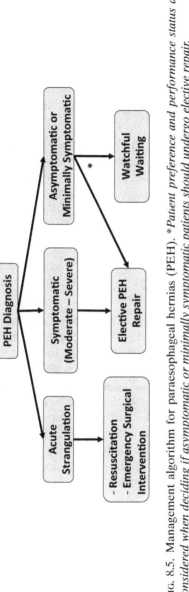

Fig. 8.5. Management algorithm for paraesophageal hernias (PEH). *Patient preference and performance status are considered when deciding if asymptomatic or minimally symptomatic patients should undergo elective repair.

**Surgery in asymptomatic or minimally symptomatic patients**

- Controversial—watchful waiting vs. elective repair of all PEH irrespective of symptoms
- Annual risk of acute strangulation: 1.1 %; mortality of elective laparoscopic PEH repair: 1.4 % [7]

  - Although this reported rate of post-PEH mortality is significantly higher than most recent surgical series (<1 %)

- Patient preference and performance status are considered when deciding if these patients should undergo elective repair. Currently elective repair is recommended in most patients of good performance status.

**Complications**

- Recurrence: Despite high anatomic recurrence on follow-up imaging after laparoscopic PEH repair (up to 50 %), the majority of patients have minor/small recurrences that remain minimally symptomatic or asymptomatic [8].

  - Patients complaining of recurrent dysphagia, heartburn, or regurgitation should be reevaluated with an upper GI study and esophagogastroscopy to assess for recurrence, excessively tight fundoplication, or slipped wrap.
  - Recurrences causing significant quality-of-life impairment and slipped wraps should be treated operatively.
  - Dysphagia is not an infrequent early consequence after the repair of large PEH due to tissue edema. Although the majority of cases resolve, endoscopic balloon dilatation can be considered after 6 weeks for persistent symptoms.

- Gastroparesis: Patients present with postoperative bloating. Evaluation is performed using gastric emptying study and esophagogastroscopy to rule out cancer and other pathologies—trial of pro-motility agents for persistent major bloating symptoms.

**Use of Prosthetic Mesh (Biologic or Synthetic)**

- Synthetic mesh: Associated with complications, such as esophageal erosion, stricture, and ulceration, requiring re-operation for mesh removal and a non-insignificant risk of esophageal resection.
- Biologic mesh: Not associated with the complications related to the use of synthetic mesh.
- Several studies have looked at outcomes of mesh reinforcement compared to primary repair of PEHs (Table 8.2).

  - Most studies that show decreased PEH recurrence rates after repair with biologic mesh either lack long-term patient follow-up or are retrospective chart reviews prone to bias.
  - One randomized trial with long-term data has been done, showing equivalent recurrence rates and complications between the use of biologic mesh and primary repair of PEHs [9].

- Despite the decreased recurrence rate with the use of synthetic mesh, they are associated with significant complications requiring re-operation and are typically not used.
- *Take-home message*: Primary repair, preferably without mesh reinforcement (biologic or synthetic), is the current standard of care.

# Motility Disorders

## *Primary Motility Disorder (Table 8.3)*

- Continuum of hypomotile and hypermotile dysfunction
- Manometry: Gold standard for diagnosis (Fig. 8.6)
- Endoscopy and contrast esophagogram as adjuncts, and to evaluate for esophagitis or cancer

TABLE 8.2. Outcomes of mesh reinforcement compared to primary repair of paraesophageal hernia repair.

| Study | Methodology | Median follow-up (months) | Recurrence | Mesh-related complications |
|---|---|---|---|---|
| **Synthetic mesh** | | | | |
| Frantzides et al. (2002) [23] | RCT: PR (N=36) vs. PTFE (36) | 31 | PR=22 %; PTFE=0 % p<0.006 | 0 % |
| Zaninotto et al. (2007) [24] | Retrospective chart review PR (N=19) vs. Goretex (35) | 71 | PR=42 %; PTFE=9 % p=0.01 | 3 % |
| **Biologic mesh** | | | | |
| Ringley et al. (2006) [25] | Prospective non-randomized PR (N=22) vs.AlloDerm (N=22) | 10 | PR=9 %; PTFE=0 % (no statistical analysis) | 0 % |
| Jacobs et al. (2007) [26] | Retrospective chart review PR (N=93) vs. Goretex (127) | PR=46 Surgisis=38 | PR=20 %; Surgisis=3 % p<0.01 | 0 % |
| Oelschlager et al. (2011) [9] | RCT: PR (N=57) vs. Surgisis (51) | 58 | PR=59 %; Surgisis=54 % p=0.7 | 0 % |

*PR* primary repair, *RCT* randomized-controlled trial, *PTFE* polytetrafluoroethylene

TABLE 8.3. Summary of pathophysiology and presentation of primary esophageal motility disorders.

| | Normal | Achalasia | Hypertensive LES | Diffuse esophageal spasm | Nutcracker esophagus | Ineffective esophageal motility |
|---|---|---|---|---|---|---|
| Clinical presentation | | • Dysphagia<br>• Weight loss<br>• Regurgitation (undigested food)<br>• Choking | • Dysphagia | • Chest pain (mimic angina)<br>• Dysphagia (intermittent, nonprogressive)<br>• Other GI functional disorders | • Chest pain (severe post-swallowing)<br>• Dysphagia<br>• Odynophagia<br>• Psychiatric disorders | • Chest pain<br>• Dysphagia<br>• Heartburn |
| Upper GI study | | • Bird's beak<br>• Dilated distal esophagus, air-fluid levels<br>• No gastric air bubble | • Dilated distal esophagus | • Corkscrew esophagus<br>• Pseudo-diverticulitis | • Normal | • Slow transit<br>• Incomplete emptying |
| LES pressure | • 15–25 mmHg | • Hypertensive (>26 mmHg) | • Hypertensive (>26 mmhg) | • Normal or elevated | • Normal | • Normal or low |
| LES relaxation | • Follows swallowing | • Incomplete | • Normal | • Normal | • Normal | • Normal |

| | | | | | |
|---|---|---|---|---|---|
| Amplitude | 50–120 mmHg | *Decreased (<40 mmHg)* | Normal | *Hypertensive (>120 mmHg)* | *Hypertensive (>200 mmHg; ~400 mmHg common)* | *Decreased (<30 mmHg)* |
| Contraction | Progressive | *Uncoordinated Simultaneous* | Normal | Simultaneous Multi-peaked *Long duration* | Long duration | Uncoordinated |
| Peristalsis | None | None | *Normal* | None | *Hypertensive peristalsis* | Abnormal |

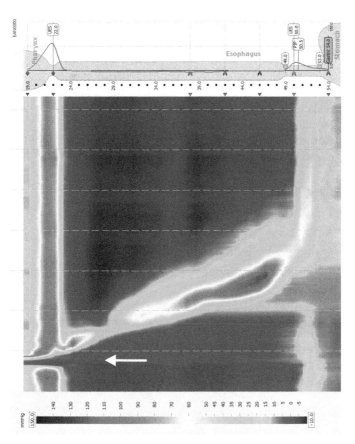
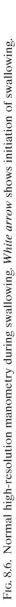

FIG. 8.6. Normal high-resolution manometry during swallowing. *White arrow* shows initiation of swallowing.

## Secondary Motility Disorders

- Systemic disorders, such as collagen vascular disorders, scleroderma, diabetes mellitus, amyloidosis, neuromuscular diseases, and Chagas' disease.

## Achalasia

**Pathophysiology**

- Myenteric plexus ganglion cell degeneration, resulting in loss of inhibitory activity, lack of peristalsis, failure of LES relaxation during swallowing, and stasis of food in the esophagus
- Results in esophageal dilation and non-peristaltic, simultaneous contractions of the esophagus

**Classification [10]:**

- Type 1 (classic):
  - Absent peristalsis with minimal esophageal pressurization (low amplitude)
  - Incomplete LES relaxation

- Type 2:
  - Absent peristalsis
  - Intermittent panesophageal pressurization (esophageal compression)
  - Incomplete LES relaxation
  - Best response to treatment (see **Management**)

- Type 3:
  - No normal peristalsis
  - Well-defined, lumen-obliterating, spastic contractions in the distal esophagus (preserved fragments of distal peristalsis or premature (spastic) contraction)
  - Incomplete LES relaxation
  - Worst response to treatment

- Functional obstruction with some preserved peristalsis
- *Vigorous Achalasia*: Outdated term used to refer to a variant form of achalasia with simultaneous pressurizations and high amplitude of contractions in response to swallowing

  - Encompasses both Type 2 and 3
  - Imprecise term because responsiveness to treatment for Types 2 and 3 is at opposite ends of the spectrum (Type 2: best response to therapy; Type 3: worse response to therapy)
  - Frequently associated with chest pain
  - Previously presumed to represent an earlier/more treatable form of achalasia; however the evidence is very limited and no consensus exists on its definition or clinical implications

**Complications:**

- Aspiration pneumonia, lung abscess, bronchiectasis
- Esophageal squamous cell carcinoma:

  - Food stasis → bacterial overgrowth → elevated nitrosamines, chronic inflammation, dysplasia
  - Prevalence 3 %; 16–33 relative risk for esophageal cancer [11]

- Esophageal adenocarcinoma:

  - Long-term reflux, chronic irritation likely due to successful interventional procedures to dilate LES
  - 8 % prevalence Barrett's esophagus [12]

**Diagnosis**

- Upper GI contrast study (Fig. 8.7):

  - Frequently demonstrates typical "bird's beak" tapering of distal esophagus with or without dilated esophagus
  - May progress to sigmoid esophagus in late stages of the disease

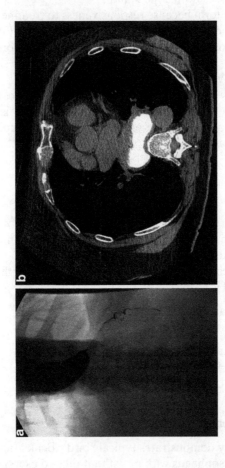

Fig. 8.7. (a) Upper GI contrast study of an achalasia patient demonstrating a typical "bird's beak" tapering of the distal esophagus. (b) CT scan shows obstruction of the distal esophagus.

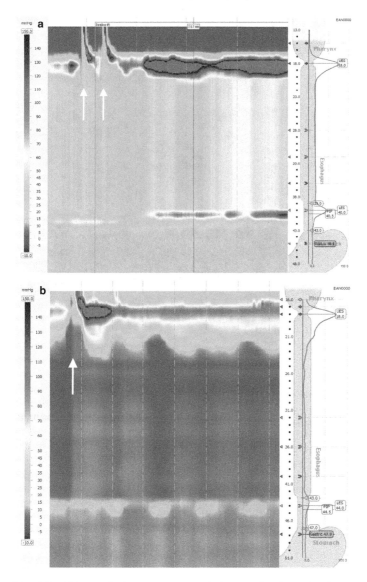

FIG. 8.8. High-resolution manometry during swallowing of patients with achalasia (**a**), scleroderma (**b**), and hypotensive lower esophageal sphincter with a hiatal hernia (**c**). *White arrows* show initiation of swallowing.

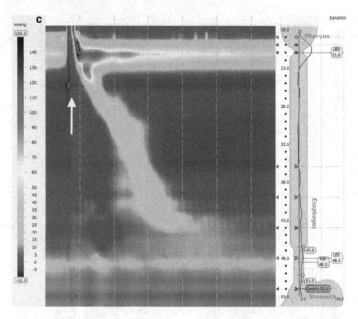

FIG. 8.8. (continued)

- Endoscopy:
  - Required in all suspected cases to rule out mechanical causes of dysphagia (especially cancer)
  - Frequently have retained secretions, candida infections, and slight resistance at esophago-gastric junction
- Manometry (Fig. 8.8):
  - Gold standard—required prior to treatment
  - Currently performed as high-resolution manometry

**Management (Fig. 8.9):**

- Goal: Relieve obstruction caused by LES—no treatment to date addresses decreased esophageal motility

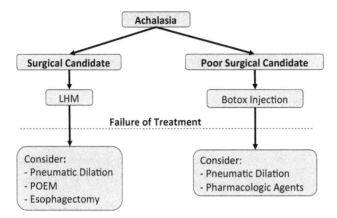

FIG. 8.9. Management algorithm for achalasia.

- Medical:

  - Short term, lack of efficacy, and high rates of side effects
  - Nitroglycerin (sublingual), nitrates, calcium channel blockers, beta-blockers

- Endoscopic:

  - Bougie dilatation

    Short-term, if any, relief of symptoms; not recommended

  - Volume-limited, pressure-controlled pneumatic balloon dilatation (PD)

    Requires large balloon at high pressures (e.g., 30–40 mm at 12 PSI)
    60 % effectiveness per dilation; 90 % after multiple dilation [13]
    4–7 % perforation risk

  - Botox (botulinum toxin) injection into LES

    Highly effective (symptom relief or improvement in up to 75–80 %) but with very limited duration
    Symptom recurrence >50 % within 6 months

Scarring due to submucosal fibrosis caused by botox injection may increase likelihood of mucosal injury if performed prior to a surgical myotomy

Usually reserved for patients of poor performance status who would not tolerate surgery

- Per-Oral Endoscopic Myotomy

Promising new procedure, however technically demanding, long learning curve

Endoscopic procedure resulting in division of the circular layer of the muscularis propria after mucosal incision

No antireflux procedure—high rates of posttreatment reflux (50 %)

Benefit over surgical myotomy is controversial

- Surgical:

  - Esophagomyotomy (Heller myotomy) standard of care for achalasia—safest and most effective

    Performed with antireflux procedure (e.g., Toupet, Dor fundoplication) to restore barrier to reflux and decrease postoperative GERD symptoms

    - Reduction of postoperative reflux from 31 to 9 % [14]
    - Highly beneficial for patients with significantly impaired esophageal motility

    Laparoscopic Heller myotomy (LHM): Shorter hospital stay, decreased postoperative pain, and improved symptoms of dysphagia and heartburn than either the open or minimally invasive transthoracic approach

    Complications: Esophageal leak (*See* Chap. 8*: Benign Esophageal Disorders (Esophageal Perforation))*, pneumothorax (opening of parietal pleura), persistent dysphagia (technical errors such as short myotomy, tight fundoplication), recurrent dysphagia (fibrosis of distal portion of myotomy), GERD (25 %)

- LHM vs. pneumatic dilation (PD) RCT meta-analyses:

    86 % (LHM) vs. 76 % (PD) 1-year response rate (OR 1.98, p = 0.02) [15]
    LHM also shown to be superior at 24 months (OR 5.06, 95 % CI 2.61–9.80) and 60 months (OR 29.83, 95 % CI 3.96–224) [16]
    PD: 4.8 % esophageal perforation rate vs. 0.6 % LHM mucosal tear rate

- LHM vs. per-oral endoscopic myotomy (POEM): Comparable safety and efficacy [17]; however long-term data for POEM are lacking and fundoplication is not done; therefore patients require long-term PPI therapy

    Approximately half of patients undergoing POEM will experience GERD or esophagitis (similar to patients undergoing LHM without fundoplication) [18]

- Esophagectomy

    Rarely required
    Indications for resection: Symptomatic patients with megaesophagus, sigmoid esophagus, and failure of esophagomyotomy

## Diffuse Esophageal Spasm

**Pathophysiology:**

- Hypermotility, muscular hypertrophy, neuronal degeneration of inhibitory branches of the myenteric plexus
- Repetitive, simultaneous, high-amplitude esophageal contractions

**Management**

- Poor overall results
- Nonsurgical:

    - Pharmacologic and endoscopic intervention as mainstay treatments

- Nitrates, calcium channel blockers, sedatives, and anticholinergics show some effectiveness
- Surgical:
  - Indications—recurrent and incapacitating symptoms, refractory to nonsurgical management, pulsion diverticula in the thoracic esophagus
  - Long esophagomyotomy via laparoscopic or thoracoscopic approach with antireflux procedure; 80 % symptom response rate

## Nutcracker Esophagus

### Pathophysiology

- Hypermotility disorder; "super-squeeze" esophagus with hypertensive (high-amplitude) peristalsis

### Management

- Nonsurgical: Mainstay treatment is pharmacologic
  - Not curative, only for symptom control
  - Anticholinergics, nitrates, calcium channel blockers, antispasmodics used for relief during acute episodes; antidepressants
- Surgical: Esophagomyotomy not shown to be beneficial

## Hypertensive LES

### Pathophysiology

- Elevated LES pressure with incomplete relaxation during swallowing; manometry inconsistent with achalasia

### Management

- Similar to achalasia
- Balloon dilation and LHM + partial fundoplication shown to have very good results for symptom relief

## *Ineffective Esophageal Motility*

### Pathophysiology

- Contraction abnormality of distal esophagus; dampened motility with low-amplitude contractions
- Poor acid clearance; high association with GERD; high acid exposure → secondary inflammation

### Management

- Prevention: Appropriate management of GERD

# Esophageal Diverticula

- Thought to be the result of primary esophageal motor disturbances or abnormalities of the LES or UES
- Can occur anywhere in the esophagus: Pharyngoesophageal, midesophageal, epiphrenic

*True diverticulum*: Involves all layers of the esophageal wall (mucosa, submucosa, and muscularis)

- Also called "*traction diverticula*," caused by external inflammatory mediastinal lymph nodes which adhere to the esophagus, especially from tuberculosis and histoplasmosis

*False diverticulum:* Only includes mucosa and submucosa

- Also called "*pulsion diverticula*" caused by increased intraluminal pressures secondary to motility abnormality in the esophagus (distal to the diverticulum), causing herniation of mucosa and submucosa through an area weakness in the esophageal musculature

## *Pharyngoesophageal (Zenker's) Diverticulum*

- Most common esophageal diverticula
- False diverticulum secondary to high resting tone from fibrosis of the cricopharyngeus muscle

- Arises proximal to UES, in Killian's triangle (area of weakness) in the posterior hypopharynx, between crico-pharyngeus muscle and inferior constrictors (Fig. 8.1)

**Clinical Presentation**

- Wide range of symptoms, depending on the size of diverticulum:

  - Asymptomatic
  - Sensation of food stuck in the throat
  - Intermittent dysphagia
  - Audible gurgling during swallowing
  - Halitosis
  - Regurgitation of undigested food
  - Cough
  - Recurrent aspiration

- Diagnosis confirmed by contrast study (lateral views permit visualization of the diverticulum posteriorly; Fig. 8.10)

**Treatment**

- Management is reserved for symptomatic patients
- Disrupting the cricopharyngeal muscle (alleviation of obstruction) is the primary goal of therapy irrespective of approach (open vs. trans-oral)
- Traditionally using an open approach through the left neck; however endoscopic repair is becoming increasingly popular. Repair includes both myotomy of the cricopha-ryngeus and obliteration of the reservoir
- Open repair (success rate >95 %):

  1. Myotomy of the proximal and distal thyropharyngeus and cricopharyngeus muscles
  2. Address the diverticulum with either a resection or pexy (preferred—avoids risk of staple line leak)

- Endoscopic procedure (success rate 80–95 %):

  - The common wall between the esophagus and diverticu-lum is divided with stapler or electrosurgery (including the distal cricopharyngeus), creating a common channel between the two (Fig. 8.11)

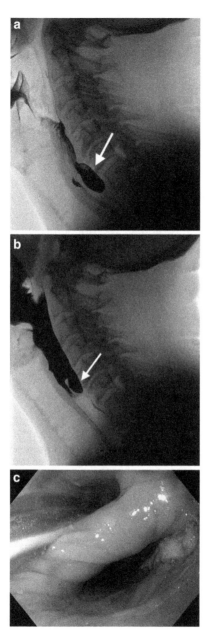

FIG. 8.10. Upper GI contrast study (**a**, **b**) and endoscopic view (**c**) showing a Zenker's diverticulum (*white arrow*).

- Can be performed with a rigid trans-oral retractor, or more recently through a standard gastroscope with en electrosurgery needle knife (Fig. 8.11)
- Risk of incomplete myotomy increased with smaller diverticula (<3 cm); therefore this method is optimal for large diverticula

- Open vs. Endoscopic [19]:

  - <3 cm: Open repair superior to endoscopic repair for symptomatic relief
  - >3 cm: Similar rates of symptomatic relief, decreased hospital stay, and faster oral intake with endoscopic approach

## Midesophageal Diverticulum

- Mostly traction diverticulum
- Usually found near the tracheal bifurcation, due to mediastinal inflammation (e.g., TB)
- Majority are asymptomatic and often an incidental finding on esophagogram, CT chest, endoscopic evaluation, and manometry to identify primary motor disorders
- Rarely require treatment

## Epiphrenic Diverticulum

- Mostly pulsion diverticulum arising cephalad to the esophago-gastric junction (Fig. 8.12)
- Almost all have some form of esophageal motility disorder—40 % of which is achalasia [20]
- Irrespective of the type of motility disorder—all symptomatic patients undergo the same approach:

  - LHM and resection of epiphrenic diverticulum

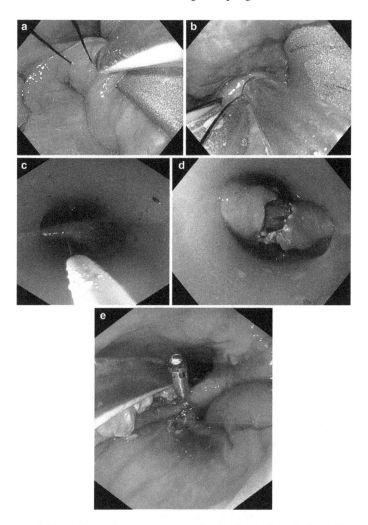

FIG. 8.11. Endoscopic management of a Zenker's diverticulum. The common wall between the esophagus and diverticulum is divided to create a common channel between the two. This can be achieved either using stapler (**a–b**) or electrosurgery (**c–e**). When using a stapler, a Weerda retractor is used to retract the pharynx and provide exposure to the diverticulum (**a**). Once the nasogastric tube is placed in the esophagus and a suture is placed through the cricopharynx (**a**), a stapler is fired (**b**) to create a common channel between the esophagus and diverticulum.

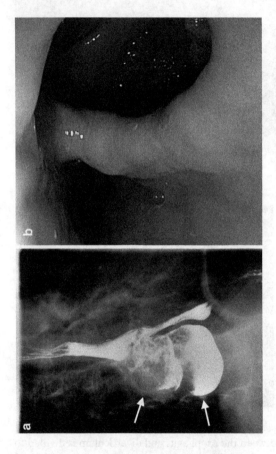

FIG. 8.12. Upper GI contrast study (**a**) and endoscopic view (**b**) of two large epiphrenic diverticula (*white arrows*) in a patient with achalasia.

# Esophageal Perforation

- Multiple etiologies (Table 8.4)
  - Iatrogenic is presently the most common (e.g., endoscopic procedures)
  - Trauma and spontaneous (either from barotrauma or malignancy) are more rare but associated with higher risk of mortality.
- May occur in the neck (most common site in iatrogenic), chest, and abdomen
- Mortality: Up to 50 % — highest for spontaneous intrathoracic perforations
- Early diagnosis and treatment <24 h decrease mortality to 7 % (20 % for >24 h; RR 2.2, 95 % CI 1.6–3.2) [21]

## Clinical Presentation and Work-Up

- Neck/substernal/epigastric pain, vomiting, and subcutaneous emphysema (Mackler's triad)

TABLE 8.4. Differential diagnosis of esophageal perforation.

| |
|---|
| *Iatrogenic* |
|   Endoscopy |
|   Dilatation |
|   Endotracheal intubation |
|   Nasogastric tube |
|   Laser therapy |
|   Surgery in the neck, chest, or abdomen |
| *Non-iatrogenic* |
|   Barotrauma (postemetic/Boerhaave's syndrome, blunt trauma, labor, convulsions, defecation) |
|   Distal obstruction |
|   Penetrating trauma |
|   Corrosive injury |
|   Infection |
|   Foreign body |

- Hematemesis, dysphagia, odynophagia
  - Cervical perforation: Neck pain, stiffness from prevertebral space infection
  - Thoracic perforation: Shortness of breath, chest pain, pneumomediastinum/pneumopericardium
- Signs of sepsis and mediastinitis
- Diagnostic modalities include CT chest/abdomen with oral contrast, endoscopy, barium contrast study
- Perforations secondary to benign etiology are usually the result of vigorous retching (Boerhaave's syndrome) and are located in the distal esophagus proximal to GEJ
  - Perforations in the thoracic or cervical esophagus are rare
- Iatrogenic endoscopic injuries occur commonly in the cervical esophagus, but can also occur at the site of therapeutic interventions (e.g., dilation, ablation, resection).

**Management (Fig. 8.13)**

- Principles of management for all patients:
  - Early and aggressive resuscitation
  - Antibiotics
  - No oral intake
  - Nutritional support
  - Source control (e.g., wide drainage of contamination)

**Contained Perforations (On Contrast Study or CT Scan):**

- If no signs of systemic inflammation, they can be managed nonoperatively with nil per os, IV antibiotics, and close surveillance
- A subset of iatrogenic perforations immediately identified can be closed using endoscopic clips and/or stents
- All others require operative intervention

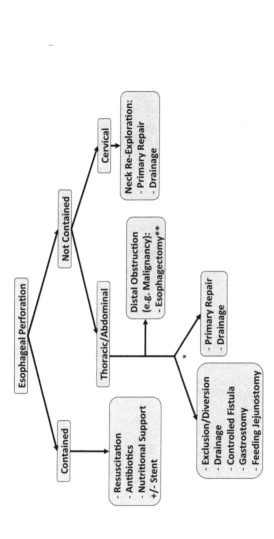

FIG. 8.13. Management algorithm for esophageal perforations. *The decision to perform primary anastomosis vs. diversion and delayed reconstruction is based on the likelihood of anastomotic breakdown (e.g., degree of inflammation, patient stability, use of vasopressors, tension on the anastomosis) **Esophagectomy can either be followed by primary repair or diversion and delayed reconstruction.

**Uncontained Perforations**

- Significantly higher mortality rate when treated conservatively (55 %) compared to surgical management (8 %) [22]

**Operative Approach**

- Intraoperative endoscopy to identify exact location of perforation as well as to rule out associated esophageal pathology (e.g., malignancy that may require resection).
- The approach to repair the perforation depends on the location of the injury on endoscopy:
  - 15–20 cm—cervical incision
  - 20–30 cm—right thoracotomy
  - 30 cm—EGJ—left thoracotomy (most common)
- Wide mediastinal drainage
- Repair defect in two layers +/− buttress
- Nutritional support (e.g., feeding jejunostomy)

# Caustic Injury

- *Population at risk:* Children, psychiatric patients, substance abuse
- Common agents: Drain cleaners, cleaning products, batteries
- Acid ingestion:
  - Immediate burning of the oral cavity, limiting ingestion, and injury
  - Pathogenesis: Coagulative necrosis with limited tissue penetration from protective eschar and limited ingestion due to immediate pain

- Alkali ingestion
  - Injury is more severe with considerable long-term sequelae
  - Pathogenesis: Liquefactive necrosis with deep tissue penetration

TABLE 8.5. Phases of injury after esophageal caustic injuries.

| Phase | Tissue injury | Onset | Duration | Inflammatory response |
|---|---|---|---|---|
| 1 | Acute necrosis | 1–4 days | 1–4 days | Intracellular protein coagulation |
| 2 | Ulceration and granulation | 3–10 days | 3–12 days | Tissue sloughing, granulation of ulcerated tissue bed *Esophagus most vulnerable to perforation* (no endoscopy or dilatation during this phase) |
| 3 | Cicatrization and scarring | 3 weeks | 1–6 months | Adhesion formation, scarring, strictures (wound contracture) Dilatation for strictures |

- Both forms of injuries can induce laryngeal and tracheo-bronchial injuries.
- Phases of injury are summarized in Table 8.5.

## Work-Up

- Urgent esophagogastroduodenoscopy

## Management

- See Table 8.6 for management of esophageal caustic injuries

### Contraindications

- Acid/base neutralization creates an exothermic reaction, worsening the injury
- Emesis or blind insertion of a nasogastric tube should be avoided to prevent perforation of necrotic esophagus or stomach.

TABLE 8.6. Management of esophageal caustic injuries.

| Grade | Description | Management |
|-------|-------------|------------|
| 1st degree | Mucosal hyperemia, edema | Observation ×24–48 h, aggressive resuscitation, acid suppression, antibiotics, nutritional support (start oral feeds once odynophagia resolves), repeat endoscopies |
| 2nd degree | Limited hemorrhage, exudate, ulceration, pseudomembranes 2A: Superficial ulcers, bleeding, exudates 2B: Deep focal or circumferential ulcers | Similar to 1st degree Patients should be monitored and reevaluated for deterioration → surgery |
| 3rd degree | Mucosal sloughing, deep ulcerations, massive hemorrhage, complete luminal obstruction, charring, perforation 3A: Focal necrosis 3B: Extensive necrosis | Aggressive resuscitation, antibiotics, acid suppression Surgical exploration, esophagogastrectomy (either primary anastomosis or diversion and controlled fistula with delayed reconstruction), gastrostomy, feeding jejunostomy |

## Surveillance

- All patients should be followed for long term due to increased risk of esophageal cancer (1,000-fold greater risk) and to manage strictures (>70 % in grades 2B/3)

# References

1. Wileman SM et al. Medical versus surgical management for gastro-oesophageal reflux disease (GORD) in adults. Cochrane Database Syst Rev. 2010;3, CD003243.
2. Katz PO, Gerson LB, Vela MF. Guidelines for the diagnosis and management of gastroesophageal reflux disease. Am J Gastroenterol. 2013;108(3):308–28. quiz 329.

3. Strate U et al. Laparoscopic fundoplication: Nissen versus Toupet two-year outcome of a prospective randomized study of 200 patients regarding preoperative esophageal motility. Surg Endosc. 2008;22(1):21–30.
4. Zornig C et al. Nissen vs Toupet laparoscopic fundoplication. Surg Endosc. 2002;16(5):758–66.
5. Ferri LE et al. Should laparoscopic paraesophageal hernia repair be abandoned in favor of the open approach? Surg Endosc. 2005;19(1):4–8.
6. Swanstrom LL et al. Esophageal motility and outcomes following laparoscopic paraesophageal hernia repair and fundoplication. Am J Surg. 1999;177(5):359–63.
7. Stylopoulos N, Gazelle GS, Rattner DW. Paraesophageal hernias: operation or observation? Ann Surg. 2002;236(4):492–500. discussion 500-1
8. Oelschlager BK et al. Laparoscopic paraesophageal hernia repair: defining long-term clinical and anatomic outcomes. J Gastrointest Surg. 2012;16(3):453–9.
9. Oelschlager BK et al. Biologic prosthesis to prevent recurrence after laparoscopic paraesophageal hernia repair: long-term follow-up from a multicenter, prospective, randomized trial. J Am Coll Surg. 2011;213(4):461–8.
10. Pandolfino JE et al. Achalasia: a new clinically relevant classification by high-resolution manometry. Gastroenterology. 2008;135(5):1526–33.
11. Leeuwenburgh I et al. Long-term esophageal cancer risk in patients with primary achalasia: a prospective study. Am J Gastroenterol. 2010;105(10):2144–9.
12. O'Neill OM, Johnston BT, Coleman HG. Achalasia: A review of clinical diagnosis, epidemiology, treatment and outcomes. World J Gastroenterol. 2013;19(35):5806–12.
13. Hulselmans M et al. Long-term outcome of pneumatic dilation in the treatment of achalasia. Clin Gastroenterol Hepatol. 2010;8(1):30–5.
14. Campos GM et al. Endoscopic and surgical treatments for achalasia: a systematic review and meta-analysis. Ann Surg. 2009;249(1):45–57.
15. Yaghoobi M et al. Laparoscopic Heller's myotomy versus pneumatic dilation in the treatment of idiopathic achalasia: a meta-analysis of randomized, controlled trials. Gastrointest Endosc. 2013;78(3):468–75.

16. Schoenberg MB et al. Laparoscopic Heller myotomy versus endoscopic balloon dilatation for the treatment of achalasia: a network meta-analysis. Ann Surg. 2013;258(6):943–52.
17. Bhayani NH, Kurian AA, Dunst CM, Sharata AM, Rieder E, Swanstrom LL. A comparative study on comprehensive, objective outcomes of laparoscopic Heller myotomy with per-oral endoscopic myotomy (POEM) for achalasia. Ann Surg. 2014; 259(6):1098–103.
18. Swanstrom LL et al. Long-term outcomes of an endoscopic myotomy for achalasia: the POEM procedure. Ann Surg. 2012; 256(4):659–67.
19. Gutschow CA et al. Management of pharyngoesophageal (Zenker's) diverticulum: which technique? Ann Thorac Surg. 2002;74(5):1677–82. discussion 1682-3.
20. Nehra D et al. Physiologic basis for the treatment of epiphrenic diverticulum. Ann Surg. 2002;235(3):346–54.
21. Biancari F et al. Current treatment and outcome of esophageal perforations in adults: systematic review and meta-analysis of 75 studies. World J Surg. 2013;37(5):1051–9.
22. Lin Y, Jiang G, Liu L, Jiang JX, Chen L, Zhao Y, et al. Management of thoracic esophageal perforation. World J Surg. 2014;38(5):1093–9.
23. Frantzides CT et al. A prospective, randomized trial of laparoscopic polytetrafluoroethylene (PTFE) patch repair vs simple cruroplasty for large hiatal hernia. Arch Surg. 2002; 137(6):649–52.
24. Zaninotto G et al. Objective follow-up after laparoscopic repair of large type III hiatal hernia. Assessment of safety and durability. World J Surg. 2007;31(11):2177–83.
25. Ringley CD et al. Laparoscopic hiatal hernia repair with human acellular dermal matrix patch: our initial experience. Am J Surg. 2006;192(6):767–72.
26. Jacobs M et al. Use of surgisis mesh in laparoscopic repair of hiatal hernias. Surg Laparosc Endosc Percutan Tech. 2007;17(5):365–8.

# Chapter 9
# Oesophageal Cancer

**Amin Madani, Sara Najmeh, and Abdullah Aloraini**

## Barrett's Oesophagus

### Overview

- Definition: Replacement of normal squamous mucosa by metaplastic columnar epithelium

    - *Any length* of columnar epithelium in the oesophagus with histological signs of *intestinal metaplasia*
    - Differs from gastric histology by presence of oesophageal musculature, lack of peritoneal covering and typical oesophageal mucous glands

- Pre-malignant condition for oesophageal adenocarcinoma (Fig. 9.1)
- Risk factors: Chronic gastroesophageal reflux disease (GERD; worse with nocturnal symptoms), risk factors for

A. Madani, M.D.
Department of Surgery, McGill University Health Center,
Montreal, QC, Canada

S. Najmeh, M.D. (✉) • A. Aloraini
Division of Surgery, McGill University Health Center,
Montreal, QC, Canada
e-mail: sara.najmeh@mail.mcgill.ca

A. Madani et al. (eds.), *Pocket Manual of General Thoracic Surgery*, DOI 10.1007/978-3-319-17497-6_9,
© Springer International Publishing Switzerland 2015

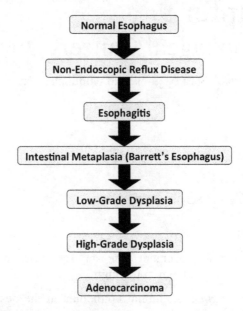

Fig. 9.1. Natural history of Barrett's oesophagus.

GERD (age, male, obesity, caffeine, alcohol, tobacco and spicy, fatty and acidic foods, visceral fat, Caucasian)

- Prevalence: 2 % in Western countries; 6–12 % of all patients undergoing oesophagogastroduodenoscopy (EGD) [1]

## Classification

- Short-segment Barrett's: ≤3 cm
- Long-segment Barrett's: >3 cm; higher risk of dysplasia and cancer [2]
- Prague Classification of Barrett's (endoscopic grading) [3]:

  – C: Circumferential extent in cm
  – M: Maximum extent in cm
  – For example, patient with 7 cm length of columnar lined mucosa with intestinal metaplasia proximal to the gastric folds, 4 cm of which is 100 % circumferential,

and 3 additional cm of non-circumferential "islands" or "tongues" of Barrett's is represented as C4M7.

## Pathophysiology

- Pathophysiology remains unclear; however acid, bile and other reflux-related products seem to play a role
- 40-fold increased risk of oesophageal and GEJ adenocarcinomas [4]

  - 0.33–0.5 %/year from non-dysplastic Barrett's to adenocarcinoma; 0.9 %/year to high-grade dysplasia
  - Correlates with Barrett's length (0.2 %/year for short segment)

- 25-fold increase in mortality from oesophageal cancer compared to general population

### Dysplasia

- Low-grade dysplasia (LGD) increases the risk of progression to high-grade dysplasia (HGD) and adenocarcinoma
- HGD is a red flag for the development, or occult presence, of adenocarcinoma

  - Many harbor synchronous occult adenocarcinoma
  - 45–60 % develop adenocarcinoma within 5 years (5 % are >T1a) [5]

## Clinical Presentation

- Most patients are asymptomatic or manifest GERD symptoms

  - Heartburn, regurgitation, acid taste in the mouth, belching, indigestion

- Atypical GERD or laryngopharyngeal reflux disease symptoms may also be present.

  - Persistent throat clearing, persistent cough, globus sensation, hoarseness, chocking episodes

## Work-Up

- EGD may suggest Barrett's with segments of salmon-colored columnar like mucosa in the lower oesophagus (Fig. 9.2).

  - Graded according to Prague criteria [3]
  - New endoscopic imaging adjuncts to increase sensitivity of targeted biopsies: chromoendoscopy, narrow-band imaging, autofluorescence, confocal microscopy.

## Management: (Fig. 9.3)

**Medical**

- Acid-suppressive therapy (proton-pump inhibitors): symptom control

  - Regression of Barrett's: 7 %; progression of Barrett's: 41 % [6]

- Use of anti-inflammatory cyclooxygenase-2 (COX-2) inhibitors as chemoprevention is controversial

**Endoscopic**

- The choice of intervention is based on site, extent, histology and pre-malignant potential of the lesion (Table 9.1).
- Ablative therapies: Radiofrequency ablation (RFA), photodynamic therapy, argon plasma coagulation (APC), cryotherapy, laser ablation, multipolar electrocoagulation (MPEC)

  - Goal: Ablate metaplastic mucosa, with subsequent re-epithelialization with normal squamous mucosa
  - RFA preferred due to its limited risks, consistent therapeutic depth, ease of use and proven efficacy of eradication of disease [7]
  - APC and MPEC: Not as effective, greater risk of strictures and buried glands

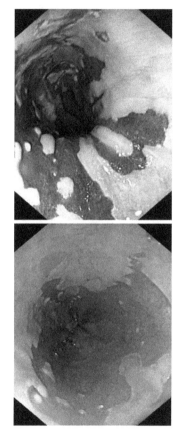

Fɪɢ. 9.2. Barrett's oesophagus is seen on oesophagogastroscopy as salmon-coloured mucosa extending from the gas-troesophageal junction.

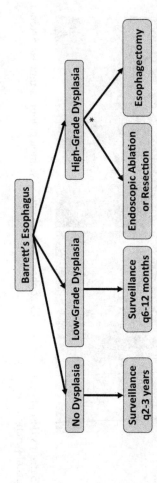

FIG. 9.3. Management algorithm for Barrett's oesophagus. *: High-grade dysplasia should be treated either endo-scopically or surgically based on several factors: *patient compliance for future endoscopic surveillance, focal vs. multifo-cal lesions, tortuous oesophagus, grade of differentiation and lymphovascular invasion if patient has associated invasive malignancy.*

TABLE 9.1. Comparison of various treatment modalities for Barrett's oesophagus.

| Procedure | Advantages | Disadvantages |
|---|---|---|
| **Endoscopic** | | |
| Ablative therapy | • Minimally invasive<br>• Ablation up to SM1<br>• Proven efficacy of eradication of dysplasia | • Operator dependant and costly<br>• Small risk of strictures/perforation<br>• Requires close follow-up and repeat endoscopies |
| Endoscopic mucosal resection | • Minimally invasive<br>• Resection up to muscularis mucosa<br>• Can be used for early localized cancer<br>• Provides pathological specimen details | • Can only resect up to 0.5–1 cm at one time (piece-meal resection for larger lesions)<br>• High rate of strictures for long-segment circumferential resections<br>• Risk of perforation<br>• Requires close follow-up and repeat endoscopies<br>• Risk of missing metachronous lesions<br>• Operator dependant and costly<br>• High risk (30 %) of local recurrence when used for early-stage oesophageal cancer [26] |
| Combined ablation/EMR | • Decreased recurrence rate compared to EMR alone | • Risk of perforation<br>• Requires close follow-up and repeat endoscopies<br>• Operator dependant and costly |
| Endoscopic submucosal dissection | • Minimally invasive<br>• Resection up to SM2/3<br>• High rates of R0 resection<br>• Can be used for early localized malignant lesions | • Limited experience<br>• Technically challenging<br>• Risk of perforation |

(continued)

TABLE 9.1. (continued)

| Procedure | Advantages | Disadvantages |
|---|---|---|
| **Surgical** | | |
| Anti-reflux surgery | • Treats the underlying cause<br>• Possible regression of metaplasia<br>• May facilitate subsequent ablative therapies | • Not proven definitively in preventing cancer in patients with Barrett's<br>• May make future surveillance difficult/inadequate |
| Oesophagectomy | • Complete resection of diseased oesophagus<br>• Provides pathological specimen details (grade, LVI, stage) | • High rates of morbidity and mortality |

Determination of the appropriate intervention should be based on site, extent, histology and pre-malignant potential of the lesion

- Most ablative therapies have an efficacy of Barrett's eradication of approximately 80–85 %. Less effective for ultra-long segments (>8 cm), tortuous oesophagus and large hiatal hernias.
- Due to high cost, usually reserved for patients with dysplastic Barrett's

- Resective therapies (Fig. 9.4)

  - Endoscopic mucosal resection (EMR)
  - Endoscopic submucosal dissection (ESD)
  - Ablative and endoscopic resection therapies are frequently used together (Fig. 9.5)
  - Endoscopic resection (EMR or ESD) is required to diagnose and possibly treat early cancers associated with Barrett's oesophagus

    This should be done for all nodular/irregular Barrett's mucosa prior to any ablative treatment
    Increases the diagnostic accuracy for occult cancer, and may be adequate oncologic treatment if an early cancer is identified

**Surgery**

- Anti-reflux surgery—controversial

  - Regression of Barrett's: 25 %; progression of Barrett's: 9 % [6]
  - Does not eliminate the risk of dysplasia and cancer
  - Laparoscopic anti-reflux surgery may be required *prior* to ablation of dysplastic Barrett's in some cases:

    Large hiatal hernias with tortuous oesophagus
    Ongoing oesophagitis despite maximal medical therapy

- Oesophagectomy

  - Reserved for HGD that is not amenable to endoscopic therapies
  - Laparoscopic oesophagectomy is the approach of choice

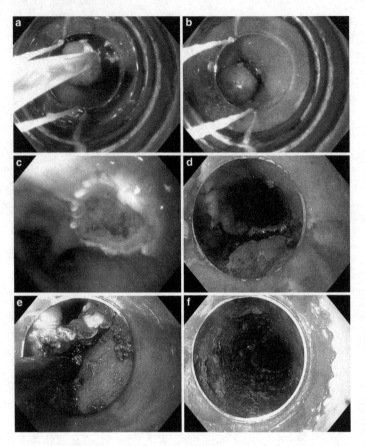

FIG. 9.4. Endoscopic resections include EMR (**a–c**) and ESD (**d–f**) for a patient with pT1aNx, moderately differentiated adenocarcinoma and no lymphovascular invasion.

# Oesophageal Cancer

## Overview

- Incidence:
  - Canada: 1,700 estimated new cases per year (nearly equivalent mortality rate)

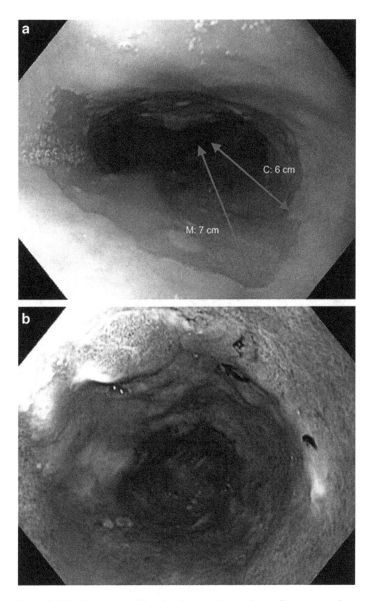

Fig. 9.5. The Prague classification is an endoscopic grading system that takes into account circumferential extent (C) and maximum extent (M). (**a**) This patient has multinodular Barrett's oesophagus C6M7. **b–c**: The extent of Barrett's can also be seen on narrow-band imaging.

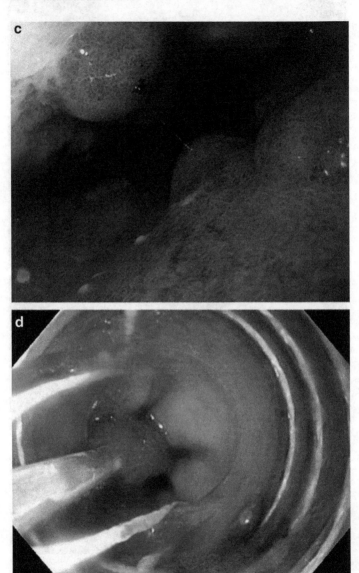

FIG. 9.5.  (continued) After undergoing EMR (**d**) confirming high-grade dysplasia and intramucosal carcinoma, the patient underwent several episodes of RFA (**e**). Finally after disease recurrence (**f**), the patient underwent a laparoscopic oesophagectomy.

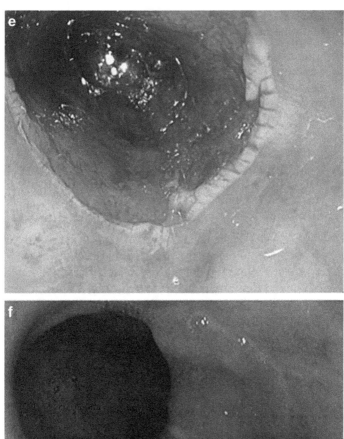

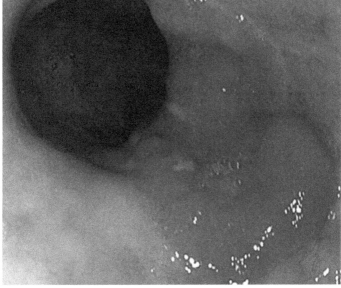

Fɪɢ. 9.5 (continued)

- USA: 18,000 estimated new cases per year (>15,000 estimated deaths) [8]

- Squamous-cell carcinoma (SCC) predominates worldwide, while in North America, adenocarcinoma represents the majority of malignancies of the oesophagus (>75 %), given the increasing incidence of Barrett's oesophagus
- SCC: Mostly upper and middle-third oesophagus
- Adenocarcinoma: Mostly middle and distal-third oesophagus and gastroesophageal junction
- Other histologic subtypes: Neuroendocrine tumour, gastrointestinal stromal tumour, adeno-squamous carcinoma, melanoma, sarcoma, lymphoma
- Risk factors:

  - SCC: Geographic location (some areas of the world are endemic), smoking, alcohol, head and neck malignancy, achalasia, caustic injury, diverticular disease, Plummer-Vinson syndrome, radiation therapy, tylosis, nitrosamines and other nitrosyl compounds
  - Adenocarcinoma: Barrett's oesophagus, GERD, obesity, smoking

## Clinical Presentation

- Most patients do not become symptomatic until late in the course of illness.
- Obstructive symptoms: Progressive dysphagia (solid food, then liquids), regurgitation, oesophageal perforation, chronic cough, aspiration
- Hematemesis, melena
- Symptoms of local invasion: Hoarseness, bronchoespohgeal fistula, empyema.
- Systemic symptoms: Weight loss, fatigue
- Physical examination may reveal cervical or supraclavicular lymph nodes

# Work-Up and Staging (Table 9.2)

- *Laboratory*: CBC, electrolytes, renal function, liver function, tumour markers (CA19-9, CEA, CA-125), total protein, albumin, pre-albumin
- *Endoscopy*: Oesophagogastroscopy (tissue diagnosis and anatomic characterization of the lesion; Fig. 9.6), endoscopic ultrasound, bronchoscopy for upper and middle-third tumours

TABLE 9.2. TNM staging classification for oesophageal cancer.

*Primary tumour (T)*

| | |
|---|---|
| T1 | Invasion of lamina propria, muscularis mucosae, submucosa |
| T1a | Invasion of lamina propria, muscularis mucosae |
| T1b | Invasion of submucosa |
| T2 | Invasion of muscularis propria |
| T3 | Invasion of adventitia |
| T4a | Invasion of pleura, pericardium or diaphragm |
| T4b | Invasion of other adjacent structures (e.g. aorta, vertebral body, trachea) |

*Regional lymph nodes (N)*

| | |
|---|---|
| N0 | No regional lymph node metastases |
| N1 | 1–2 regional lymph nodes |
| N2 | 3–6 regional lymph nodes |
| N3 | >6 regional lymph nodes |

*Distant metastasis (M)*

| | |
|---|---|
| M0 | No distant metastasis |
| M1 | Distant metastasis |

*Squamous-cell carcinoma*

| Stage | T | N | M | Grade | Tumour location |
|---|---|---|---|---|---|
| IA | T1 | N0 | M0 | 1 | Any |
| IB | T1 | N0 | M0 | 2,3 | Any |
| | T2–3 | N0 | M0 | 1 | Lower |
| IIA | T2–3 | N0 | M0 | 1 | Upper, middle |
| | T2–3 | N0 | M0 | 2,3 | Lower |
| IIB | T2–3 | N0 | M0 | 2,3 | Upper, middle |
| | T1–2 | N1 | M0 | Any | Any |

(continued)

TABLE 9.2. (continued)

| IIIA | T1–T2 | N2 | M0 | Any | Any |
|------|-------|-----|-----|-----|-----|
|  | T3 | N1 | M0 | Any | Any |
|  | T4a | N0 | M0 | Any | Any |
| IIIB | T3 | N2 | M0 | Any | Any |
| IIIC | T4a | N1, N2 | M0 | Any | Any |
|  | T4b | Any N | M0 | Any | Any |
|  | Any T | N3 | M0 | Any | Any |
| IV | Any T | Any N | M1 | Any | Any |

*Adenocarcinoma*

| Stage | *T* | *N* | *M* | *Grade* | *Tumour location* |
|-------|-----|-----|-----|---------|-------------------|
| IA | T1 | N0 | M0 | 1,2 | Any |
| IB | T1 | N0 | M0 | 3 | Any |
|  | T2 | N0 | M0 | 1,2 | Any |
| IIA | T2 | N0 | M0 | 3 | Any |
| IIB | T3 | N0 | M0 | Any | Any |
|  | T1–2 | N1 | M0 | Any | Any |
| IIIA | T1–T2 | N2 | M0 | Any | Any |
|  | T3 | N1 | M0 | Any | Any |
|  | T4a | N0 | M0 | Any | Any |
| IIIB | T3 | N2 | M0 | Any | Any |
| IIIC | T4a | N1, N2 | M0 | Any | Any |
|  | T4b | Any N | M0 | Any | Any |
|  | Any T | N3 | M0 | Any | Any |
| IV | Any T | Any N | M1 | Any | Any |

Used with permission of the American Joint Committee on Cancer (AJCC), Chicago, Illinois. The original and primary source for this information is the AJCC Cancer Staging Manual, Seventh Edition (2010) published by Springer Science + Business Media

- *Imaging*: CT chest/abdomen (Fig. 9.7), PET-CT
- *Physiologic tests*: 6-min walk test, 24-h creatinine clearance, audiology and echocardiogram for possible chemotherapy
- Multi-disciplinary tumour board discussion
- Diagnostic laparoscopy or thoracoscopy can be done at the time of operation to avoid unnecessary laparotomy or thoracotomy in approximately 20 % of patients

  - Mostly useful for bulky T3 or T4a disease to detect peritoneal or unresectable disease not seen on non-invasive staging investigations

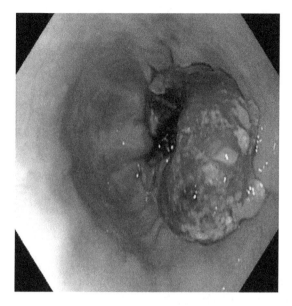

Fɪɢ. 9.6. Oesophageal adenocarcinoma seen on oesophagogastroscopy.

## Management: Localized Disease (Fig. 9.8)

- Very early disease can be effectively treated by oesophagus-sparing resection techniques with equivalent oncologic outcomes [9].
- Endoscopic therapy compared to oesophagectomy for T1a lesions is associated with lower morbidity (0 vs 39 %; $p < 0.0001$), with equivalent survival (94 % at 3 years) [10].
- Candidates for oesophagus-sparing endoscopic therapy:
  - *Localized disease with a negligible risk of lymph node metastasis (Table 9.3)*
  - *Lesion is amenable to en-bloc resection*
  - Patient compliance for surveillance
  - Absence of other significant oesophageal disorders (e.g. motility disorders, oesophagitis, large hiatal hernia, strictures)
  - Short Barrett's oesophagus

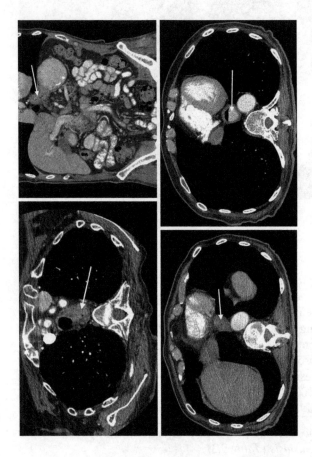

Fig. 9.7. Adenocarcinomas of the gastroesophageal junction causing obstructive symptoms. *White arrows* denote a thickened mass and a small oesophageal lumen.

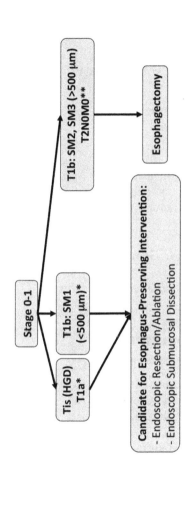

Fig. 9.8. Management algorithm for localized disease. *: Endoscopic resection is reserved for candidates who fit specific criteria. See Chap. 9: Esophageal Cancer (Criteria for Esophagus-Sparing Endoscopic Resection). **: T2N0M0 lesions are considered either stage I or II depending on grade and location. See Chap. 9: Esophageal Cancer (Management: Locally Advanced Disease).

238    A. Madani et al.

- Following endoscopic therapy, if pathology report reveals high risk for lymph node metastasis (e.g. poorly differentiated, lymphovascular invasion, depth greater than SM1), either margins should be revised or patient should undergo an oesophagectomy.

  – Otherwise endoscopic surveillance is done at 3, 6, 9 and 12 months, then annually

- High rate of failure with oesophagus-sparing endoscopic therapy:

  – Long Barrett's oesophagus (≥8 cm)
  – Poorly differentiated
  – Large size (>3 cm)
  – Ulcerations
  – Lymphovascular invasion
  – Occupying >75 % oesophageal circumference (high risk of severe strictures)

**Criteria for Oesophagus-Sparing Endoscopic Resection**

- *Well or moderately differentiated lesion:*

  – If no ulceration or elevated → no size limitation (T1a) or ≤3 cm T1b (SM1 lesion)
  – If ulceration → ≤3 cm
  – No lymphovascular invasion

- *Undifferentiated lesion:* Must have no ulceration, no lymphovascular invasion, ≤2 cm and T1a
- All lesions: No lymph node metastasis

**Risk of Lymph Node Metastasis (Table 9.3)**

- Risk of lymph node metastasis increases with depth of invasion: T1: 0–50 %; T3–T4: >80 % [11–14]

  – Tis: 0 %
  – T1a: 3–10 %
  – T1b: 25–30 % (SM1: 0–10 %; SM2/SM3: 30–50 %) [15, 16]

- Scoring system developed to predict lymph node metastasis using multivariate analysis (Table 9.3) [16]
- Strongest predictors of lymph node metastasis are [16]:
  - Lymphovascular invasion (OR 7.5, 95 % CI 3.3–17.1)
  - Tumour size (OR 1.35 per cm, 95 % CI 1.1–1.7)

## Management: Locally Advanced Disease

- Management of locally advanced disease is dependent on histopathology:

### Adenocarcinoma (Fig. 9.9)

- Patients with localized disease should undergo surgical resection (either endoscopic or oesophagectomy)
- Most patients with locally advanced disease typically undergo induction therapy with either neoadjuvant chemotherapy or chemoradiation

TABLE 9.3. Lymph node metastasis prediction scoring system developed using multivariate analysis [16].

| Lymph node metastasis prediction | |
| --- | --- |
| **Factors** | **Points** |
| Size | 1 per cm |
| Depth of Invasion | |
| • T1a | +0 |
| • T1b | +2 |
| Differentiation | |
| • Well differentiated | +0 |
| • Moderately/poorly differentiated | +3 |
| Lymphovascular Invasion (LVI) | |
| • None | +0 |
| • LVI | +6 |
| *Risk calculation* | Risk of lymph node metastasis |
| Low risk (0–1 points) | <2 % |
| Moderate risk (2–4 points) | 3–6 % |
| High risk (≥5 points) | ≥7 % |

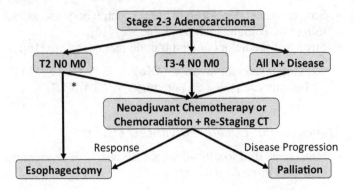

Fig. 9.9. Management algorithm for locally advanced adenocarcinoma. *: Controversial (See Chap. 9: Esophageal Cancer (Management: Locally Advanced Disease)).

- Controversy exists surrounding the management of T2N0M0 lesions: surgery vs. induction therapy + surgery

  - >85 % of clinically staged cT2N0M0 patients are incorrectly staged [17]

    Overstaged: 55 % — T1a (38 %); T1b (52 %)
    Understaged: 32 % — Node positive (76 %)

  - Management dictated by institutional protocols. Since the majority of patients are overstaged, some prefer surgery first. If patients have good performance status or bulky tumours, we tend to offer them induction therapy prior to surgery. For patients found to have been understaged after surgery, adjuvant therapy should be offered (chemoradiation according to the Intergroup 0116 Trial results) [18]

**Squamous-Cell Carcinoma (Fig. 9.10)**

- *Definitive Chemoradiation vs. Neoadjuvant Chemoradiation ± Surgery*

  - Since 40–50 % of squamous cell carcinomas have a complete pathologic response after chemoradiation [19],

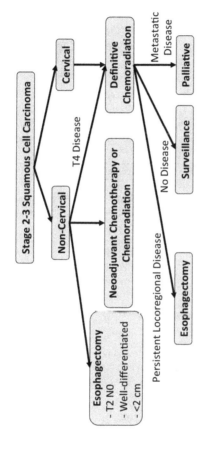

FIG. 9.10. Management algorithm for locally advanced squamous-cell carcinoma.

controversy exists regarding planned or salvage surgery for these patients.

- Mostly cervical SCC patients tend to undergo definitive chemoradiation followed by restaging. Patients with persistent disease should undergo resection, while those with a clinically complete response can undergo either surveillance (low-risk tumour, high operative risk) or resection (high-risk tumour, low operative risk).

- Two RCTs have been done showing no improvement in overall survival with surgery, despite an improvement in locoregional recurrence in SCC patients (Table 9.4). However, the operative mortality in these studies is higher than benchmark standards.

TABLE 9.4. Landmark studies comparing chemoradiation/surgery with chemoradiation alone.

| Study | Methodology | Outcomes | Toxicity + compliance |
|---|---|---|---|
| *Chemoradiation + surgery* vs. *chemoradiation* | | | |
| Bedenne et al. (2007) [27] | **RCT** CRTx + Surgery ($N=129$) CRTx ($N=130$) | **Median OS**: 18 months (CRTx + surgery), 19 months (CRTx), $p > 0.05$ **Median 2-year progression-free survival**: 66 % (CRTx + surgery), 57 % (CRTx), $p < 0.001$ | Grade $\geq 3$: 82 % Compliance: 64 % |
| Stahl et al. (2005) [28] | **RCT** CRTx + Surgery ($N=86$) CRTx ($N=86$) | **Median OS**: - 16 months (CRTx + surgery), 15 months (CRTx), $p > 0.05$ **Median 2-year progression-free survival**: 64 % (CRTx + surgery), 41 % (CRTx), $p = 0.003$ | Grade $\geq 3$: 100 % |

*RCT* randomized-controlled trial, *OS* overall survival, *CRTx* chemoradiation therapy

– *Salvage Oesophagectomy*: Resection after 90 days from completion of curative-intent chemoradiation; associated with greater morbidity compared to planned oesophagectomy after induction therapy.

## Oesophagectomy

- Oesophagectomy without induction therapy reserved for:

  – Patients who are not a candidate for oesophagus-preserving endoscopic interventions (Fig. 9.8)
  – Selected patients with T2N0M0 disease
  – Patients medically unfit to receive tri-modality therapy
  – Emergency surgery for obstruction, bleeding or perforation

- Various options available with significant variability in outcomes between individuals, institutions and trials:

  – Ivor-Lewis oesophagectomy: Distal-third, GEJ and proximal stomach tumours
  – Minimally invasive oesophagectomy (either laparoscopic/thoracoscopic or laparoscopic/thoracoscopic/cervical approach)
  – Thoracoabdominal oesophagectomy: Distal-third, GEJ and proximal stomach tumours

    Large generous surgical field, ideal for bulky GEJ (Siewert 3) tumours, and for retroperitoneal lymph nodes

  – McKeown (three-field) oesophagectomy: Upper and middle-third tumours

    Cervical anastomoses have higher anastomotic leak rate, but decreased leak-related morbidity compared to intrathoracic anastomoses. *See Chap. 2*: Peri-Operative Care of the Thoracic Patient (*Esophageal Anastomotic Leak*)

- Transhiatal oesophagectomy: Upper and middle-third tumours

  Although a thoracotomy incision is avoided, less lymph nodes are harvested using this technique

  Largely replaced by laparoscopic approaches in most high-volume centres

- A tailored approach for each patient is preferred taking into account patient and tumour factors

  - Ideal approach balances: 1) optimization of oncologic outcomes (appropriate lymph node basin dissection and R0 resection) and 2) reduces the risk of peri-operative complications.

- Reconstruction:

  - Various conduits available: Stomach, jejunum, colon
  - Stomach is the preferred conduit due to its reliable blood supply and single anastomosis.
  - Intestinal conduits require multiple anastomoses.

## Lymph Node Dissection

- NCCN guidelines recommend ≥15 lymph nodes during en-bloc oesophagectomy [20].
- Total lymph nodes harvested (>23) and negative lymph node status shown to be independent predictors of overall survival [21, 22].
- En-bloc oesophagectomy with extended lymph node dissection improves disease-free survival for patients with stages II/III/IV [23], with new data suggesting survival benefit for patients with N1 and N2 disease (1–6 regional lymph node metastases), with minimal effect for N0 and N3 disease (0 or >6 lymph nodes).

## Neoadjuvant and Adjuvant Therapy

- Resection alone for locally advanced disease is associated with low overall survival.

- Many trials have been done looking at outcomes of adjuvant and neoadjuvant therapy.

  - *Unfortunately, there are significant inconsistencies due to pooling of SCC and adenocarcinoma histologies.* Response to treatment varies significantly between these two histologies—most notably the increased radiosensitivity of SCC, which has a significantly greater pathologic complete response rate (PCR) compared to adenocarcinoma.

- While controversial, at our institution, we tend to treat similar histologies with similar treatment irrespective of location with respect to the diaphragm (i.e. distal gastric/EGJ adenocarcinoma and oesophageal adenocarcinoma).

**Induction therapy (Table 9.5):**

- Advantages:

  - Downstages tumour and improves resection margins (pathologic complete response with induction chemoradiation = 10–50 %, depending on histopathology and regimen)
  - Well tolerated with minimal morbidity compared to adjuvant therapy (patients have decreased performance status post-operatively)
  - High patient compliance (>95 % proceed to surgery)

- Strong evidence supports neoadjuvant chemoradiation and neoadjuvant chemotherapy followed by restaging and surgery as the standard of care for most patients with locally advanced (T2–4, N0–1) disease and selected patients with T2N0M0 disease.
- Post-operative complications and early mortality in patients receiving induction therapy seem to be comparable to surgery alone, despite higher risk of wound infections, transfusion requirements and longer chest tube duration [19, 24].
- Critical analysis of the results form these major studies reveals a strong response of SCC to preoperative

TABLE 9.5. Summary of evidence for induction therapy. Most landmark trials have been pooled for comparison by Sjoquist et al. in a meta-analysis [25]

| Study | Methodology | Outcomes |
|---|---|---|
| *Surgery* vs. *neoadjuvant chemoradiation + surgery* | | |

- Given the very high PCR rate for SCC (two-fold greater than adenocarcinoma), the survival data reveals that the positive results from pooled analysis are largely driven by the SCC subgroup of patients [25]
- Neoadjuvant CRTx is an acceptable standard of care for locally advanced disease with clear benefits for SCC; however it is still controversial for adenocarcinoma

| Study | Methodology | Outcomes |
|---|---|---|
| Van Hagen et al. (2012) CROSS group [19] | **RCT** CRTx + Surgery ($N=178$) Surgery ($N=188$) *AdenoCa*: 75 % *SCC*: 23 % **Regimen**: Carboplatin/ paclitaxel + 41 Gy (23 fractions) x 5 weeks | **Median OS**: <br> • 49 months (CRTx + Surgery), 24 months (Surgery) <br> • Hazard ratio: 0.66 (95 % CI 0.5–0.88, $p=0.003$) (AdenoCa: 0.74 (0.54–1.02); SCC: 0.45 (0.24–0.84)) **PCR**: 29 % (AdenoCa: 24 %; SCC: 49 %) <br> **R0 resection rate**: <br> • 92 % (CRTx + Surgery), 69 % (Surgery), $p < 0.001$ |
| Mariette et al. (2014) FFCD 9901 [29] | **RCT (early stage 1 or 2)** CRTx + Surgery ($N=98$) Surgery ($N=97$) **Regimen**: 5-FU/ cisplatin + 45 Gy (25 fractions) × 5 weeks | **3-year OS**: <br> • 48 % (CRTX + Surgery), 53 % (Surgery) <br> • Hazard ratio: 0.99 (95 % CI 0.69–1.40, $p=0.94$) <br> **Post-operative mortality**: <br> • 11 % (CRTX + Surgery), 3 % (Surgery), $p=0.049$ |
| Walsh et al. (1996) [30] | **RCT (AdenoCa)** CRTx + Surgery ($N=58$) Surgery ($N=55$) **Regimen**: 5-FU/ cisplatin + 40 Gy (15 fractions) × 3 weeks | **Median survival**: <br> • 16 months (CRTX + Surgery), 11 months (Surgery), $p=0.01$ <br> **Pathologic complete response** (after CRTX): 25 % |

(continued)

TABLE 9.5. (continued)

| Study | Methodology | Outcomes |
|---|---|---|
| *Surgery* vs. *neoadjuvant chemotherapy + surgery* | | |
| Medical Research Council Oesophageal Cancer Working Group (2002) [31] | **RCT** CRTx + Surgery ($N=400$) Surgery ($N=402$) **Regimen**: 5-FU/ cisplatin | **Overall survival**: <br>• Hazard ratio: 0.79 (95 % CI 0.67–0.93, $p=0.004$) <br>(favouring CRTx + surgery over surgery alone) |
| *Surgery* vs. *peri-operative chemotherapy + surgery* | | |
| Ychou et al. (2011) FNCLCC/ FFCD [32] | **RCT (AdenoCa)** CRTx + Surgery ($N=113$) Surgery ($N=111$) **Regimen**: 2–4 cycles 5-FU/cisplatin peri-operatively | **5-Year OS**: <br>• 38 % (CRTx + Surgery), 24 % (Surgery) <br>• Hazard ratio: 0.69 (95 % CI 0.5–0.95, $p=0.02$) <br>**5-year disease-free survival**: <br>• 34 % (CRTx + Surgery), 19 % (Surgery) <br>• Hazard ratio: 0.65 (95 % CI 0.89–0.95, $p=0.003$) <br>**R0 resection rate**: 84 % (CRTx + Surgery), 73 % (Surgery), $p<0.001$ |
| Cunningham et al. (2011) MAGIC Trial [33] | **RCT** CTx + Surgery ($N=250$) Surgery ($N=253$) **Regimen**: 3 cycles epirubicin/ cisplatin/5-FU peri-operatively | **Median OS**: <br>• Hazard ratio: 0.75 (95 % CI 0.6–0.93, $p=0.009$) <br>**Progression-free survival**: <br>• Hazard ratio: 0.66 (95 % CI 0.53–0.81, $p<0.001$) |
| Ferri et al. (2011) [34] | **Phase 2 trial** CTx + Surgery ($N=250$) **Regimen**: 3 cycles docetaxel/cisplatin/5-FU peri-operatively | **3-year overall survival**: <br>• 60 % |

(continued)

TABLE 9.5. (continued)

| Study | Methodology | Outcomes |
|-------|-------------|----------|

*Neoadjuvant chemoradiation + surgery* vs. *neoadjuvant chemotherapy + surgery*

- Direct comparisons between neoadjuvant CTx and CRTx are complicated by low accrual
- Ample literature to support either approach
- Local institutional protocols and patient histology will dictate choice of regimen

*RCT* randomized-controlled trial, *OS* overall survival, *PCR* pathologic complete response, *CRTx* chemoradiation therapy, *CTx* chemotherapy, *AdenoCa* adenocarcinoma, *SCC* squamous-cell carcinoma

chemo-radiotherapy, but less so for adenocarcinoma. Excellent results from neoadjuvant/peri-operative chemotherapy in adenocarcinoma patients from European trials make this an attractive option for this patient population.
- No clear advantage has been established to support one regimen over another. Institutional protocols are highly variable. At our institution, we use DCF regimen [docetaxel (Taxotere) 75 mg/m2 I.V. day 1, cisplatin 75 mg/m2 I.V. day 1, 5-FU 750 mg/m2 continuous infusion for 120 h, every 3 weeks] for three cycles before and after resection for adenocarcinoma patients and neoadjuvant chemo-radiotherapy (weekly Carboplatin/Taxol with concurrent 41.4 Gy external beam radiation therapy).

**Adjuvant therapy (Table 9.6):**

- Advantages: Improved patient selection based on pathologic stage, thereby avoiding unnecessary toxicity in patients who will not benefit from tri-modality therapy (e.g. cT2N0 patients)
- Associated with poor patient compliance and high-grade (≥3) toxicity
- Indications: Patients who did not receive induction therapy preoperatively (e.g. unexpected N1 disease, emergency surgery for obstruction, perforation or bleeding)

TABLE 9.6. Landmark studies comparing adjuvant chemoradiation/surgery with surgery alone.

| Study | Methodology | Outcomes | Toxicity + compliance |
|---|---|---|---|
| *Surgery vs. surgery + adjuvant chemoradiation* | | | |
| MacDonald et al. (2001) [18] | **RCT**<br>Surgery ($N=275$)<br>CRTx + Surgery ($N=281$) | **Median OS:**  27 months (surgery), 36 months (CRTx + surgery)   Hazard ratio: 1.35 (95 % CI 1.09–1.66, $p=0.005$)<br>**Median relapse-free survival:**  19 months (surgery), 30 months (CRTx + surgery)   Hazard ratio: 1.52 (95 % CI 1.23–1.86, $p<0.001$) | Grade ≥3: 82 %<br>Compliance: 64 % |
| Rice et al. (2003) [35] | **Prospective non-randomized trial**<br>Surgery ($N=52$)<br>Surgery + CRTx ($N=31$) | **Median 4-year survival:**  15 months (surgery), 28 months (CRTx + surgery), $p=0.05$<br>**Median time to recurrence:**  13 months (surgery), 25 months (CRTx + surgery), $p=0.04$<br>**Median recurrence-free survival**  10 months (surgery), 22 months (CRTx + surgery), $p=0.02$ | Grade ≥3: 100 % |

*RCT randomized-controlled trial, OS overall survival; CRTx chemoradiation therapy*

## Management: Local Recurrence

- Thorough evaluation to rule out distant metastasis
- Anastomotic recurrence normally appears in the context of advanced disease and is normally managed with radiation (locoregional) and/or chemotherapy (distant metastasis).
- Selected cases of isolated anastomotic recurrence in medically fit patients can be managed surgically.

## Metastatic Disease and Palliative Options

- Patients medically unfit for surgery can undergo either chemotherapy/chemoradiation or palliative therapy if physiologically unfit to tolerate it.
- Palliative options:
  - Tumour debulking (endoscopic or open)
  - Endoscopic stenting/dilatation
- Nutritional support: Feeding jejunostomy, gastrostomy

# References

1. Ronkainen J et al. Prevalence of Barrett's esophagus in the general population: an endoscopic study. Gastroenterology. 2005;129(6):1825–31.
2. Hirota WK et al. Specialized intestinal metaplasia, dysplasia, and cancer of the esophagus and esophagogastric junction: prevalence and clinical data. Gastroenterology. 1999;116(2):277–85.
3. Sharma P et al. The development and validation of an endoscopic grading system for Barrett's esophagus: the Prague C & M criteria. Gastroenterology. 2006;131(5):1392–9.
4. Desai TK et al. The incidence of oesophageal adenocarcinoma in non-dysplastic Barrett's oesophagus: a meta-analysis. Gut. 2012;61(7):970–6.
5. Max Almond L, Barr H. Management controversies in Barrett's oesophagus. J Gastroenterol. 2014;49(2):195–205.
6. Ortiz A et al. Conservative treatment versus antireflux surgery in Barrett's oesophagus: long-term results of a prospective study. Br J Surg. 1996;83(2):274–8.

7. Shaheen NJ et al. Radiofrequency ablation in Barrett's esophagus with dysplasia. N Engl J Med. 2009;360(22):2277–88.

8. Siegel R, Naishadham D, Jemal A. Cancer statistics, 2013. CA Cancer J Clin. 2013;63(1):11–30.

9. Pech O et al. Comparison between endoscopic and surgical resection of mucosal esophageal adenocarcinoma in Barrett's esophagus at two high-volume centers. Ann Surg. 2011;254(1):67–72.

10. Zehetner J et al. Endoscopic resection and ablation versus esophagectomy for high-grade dysplasia and intramucosal adenocarcinoma. J Thorac Cardiovasc Surg. 2011;141(1):39–47.

11. Nigro JJ et al. Prevalence and location of nodal metastases in distal esophageal adenocarcinoma confined to the wall: implications for therapy. J Thorac Cardiovasc Surg. 1999;117(1):16–23. discussion 23-5.

12. Stein HJ et al. Early esophageal cancer: pattern of lymphatic spread and prognostic factors for long-term survival after surgical resection. Ann Surg. 2005;242(4):566–73. discussion 573-5.

13. Westerterp M et al. Outcome of surgical treatment for early adenocarcinoma of the esophagus or gastro-esophageal junction. Virchows Arch. 2005;446(5):497–504.

14. Tajima Y et al. Histopathologic findings predicting lymph node metastasis and prognosis of patients with superficial esophageal carcinoma: analysis of 240 surgically resected tumors. Cancer. 2000;88(6):1285–93.

15. Ancona E et al. Prediction of lymph node status in superficial esophageal carcinoma. Ann Surg Oncol. 2008;15(11):3278–88.

16. Lee L et al. Predicting lymph node metastases in early esophageal adenocarcinoma using a simple scoring system. J Am Coll Surg. 2013;217(2):191–9.

17. Rice TW et al. T2N0M0 esophageal cancer. J Thorac Cardiovasc Surg. 2007;133(2):317–24.

18. Macdonald JS et al. Chemoradiotherapy after surgery compared with surgery alone for adenocarcinoma of the stomach or gastro-esophageal junction. N Engl J Med. 2001;345(10):725–30.

19. van Hagen P et al. Preoperative chemoradiotherapy for esophageal or junctional cancer. N Engl J Med. 2012;366(22):2074–84.

20. National Comprehensive Cancer Network Clinical Practice Guidelines in Oncology – Esophageal and Esophagogastric Junction Cancers. 2013. 2.2013.

21. Schwarz RE, Smith DD. Clinical impact of lymphadenectomy extent in resectable esophageal cancer. J Gastrointest Surg. 2007;11(11):1384–93. discussion 1393-4.

22. Peyre CG et al. The number of lymph nodes removed predicts survival in esophageal cancer: an international study on the impact of extent of surgical resection. Ann Surg. 2008;248(4):549–56.
23. Lee PC et al. Predictors of recurrence and disease-free survival in patients with completely resected esophageal carcinoma. J Thorac Cardiovasc Surg. 2011;141(5):1196–206.
24. Taylor MD et al. Induction chemoradiotherapy and surgery for esophageal cancer: survival benefit with downstaging. Ann Thorac Surg. 2013;96(1):225–30. discussion 230-1.
25. Sjoquist KM et al. Survival after neoadjuvant chemotherapy or chemoradiotherapy for resectable oesophageal carcinoma: an updated meta-analysis. Lancet Oncol. 2011;12(7):681–92.
26. Manner H et al. Early Barrett's carcinoma with "low-risk" submucosal invasion: long-term results of endoscopic resection with a curative intent. Am J Gastroenterol. 2008;103(10):2589–97.
27. Bedenne L et al. Chemoradiation followed by surgery compared with chemoradiation alone in squamous cancer of the esophagus: FFCD 9102. J Clin Oncol. 2007;25(10):1160–8.
28. Stahl M et al. Chemoradiation with and without surgery in patients with locally advanced squamous cell carcinoma of the esophagus. J Clin Oncol. 2005;23(10):2310–7.
29. Mariette C et al. Surgery alone versus chemoradiotherapy followed by surgery for stage I and II esophageal cancer: final analysis of randomized controlled phase III trial FFCD 9901. J Clin Oncol. 2014;32(23):2416–22.
30. Walsh TN et al. A comparison of multimodal therapy and surgery for esophageal adenocarcinoma. N Engl J Med. 1996;335(7):462–7.
31. Medical Research Council Oesophageal Cancer Working G. Surgical resection with or without preoperative chemotherapy in oesophageal cancer: a randomised controlled trial. Lancet. 2002;359(9319):1727–33.
32. Ychou M et al. Perioperative chemotherapy compared with surgery alone for resectable gastroesophageal adenocarcinoma: an FNCLCC and FFCD multicenter phase III trial. J Clin Oncol. 2011;29(13):1715–21.
33. Cunningham D et al. Perioperative chemotherapy versus surgery alone for resectable gastroesophageal cancer. N Engl J Med. 2006;355(1):11–20.
34. Ferri LE et al. Perioperative docetaxel, cisplatin, and 5-fluorouracil (DCF) for locally advanced esophageal and gastric adenocarcinoma: a multicenter phase II trial. Ann Oncol. 2012;23(6):1512–7.
35. Rice TW et al. Benefit of postoperative adjuvant chemoradiotherapy in locoregionally advanced esophageal carcinoma. J Thorac Cardiovasc Surg. 2003;126(5):1590–6.

# Index

A. Madani et al. (eds.), *Pocket Manual of General
Thoracic Surgery*, DOI 10.1007/978-3-319-17497-6,
© Springer International Publishing Switzerland 2015

CPSIA information can be obtained
at www.ICGtesting.com
Printed in the USA
LVHW082103030521
686351LV00010B/452

9 783319 174969